The Great Medical Controversy of our Time:

Why Vaccines MUST be Implicated in the Occurrence of Regressive Autism.

Preface

In early 2013 I was invited to submit a book chapter for inclusion in a book. This book publisher had read an article which had earlier been published in the North American Journal of Medical Sciences .....

Ewing GW. What is regressive autism and why does it occur? Is it the consequence of multi-systemic dysfunction affecting the elimination of heavy metals and the ability to regulate neural temperature? ***N.Am.J.Med.Sci.*** 2009;1(2):28-47.

.... and requested me to revise and update this article. The editorial team at the North American Journal of Medical Sciences have previously advised that this article has been widely read.

'In a recent investigation of click/citation of publication online, your published article "What is regressive autism and why does it occur? Is it the consequence of multi-systemic dysfunction affecting the elimination of heavy metals and the ability to regulate neural temperature?" ***have obtained a very high click/citation. This will tell that your publication has been read/cited at a very high number of readers.***

The North American Journal of Medical Sciences is still free of charge for submission, publication and read, which will at most exposure to every part of the world. On the other hand, your article is so interesting with a great number of readers in the world. ***We are really proud of your publications in the journal!'***

Finally, the book chapter was submitted to three reviewers for their comments. Of the three reviewers the first reviewer authorised acceptance and publication of this book chapter with little, if any, need for revision however the other two reviewers were virulently opposed to the publication of this book chapter. We include their comments in order to illustrate the disparity of opinions which are provoked by texts which dare to criticise vaccines.

Reviewer 1 commented favourably upon the article and recommended that the article be published in its current form with some minor revisions.

Reviewer 2 commented:

'This chapter fails to fully examine the counter-evidence in the literature which has examined the iatrogenic link in regressive autism and found that correlation not supported.

The whole chapter is biased towards the author's hypothesis. Studies that not supported his hypothesis are not mentioned at all. His review of the epidemiological data on autism and more special on regressive form of it, is also very biased. There's a lack of a comprehensive view of the epidemiology of autism including many very good studies published in last years.

The hypothesis of the relationship between the regressive form of autism and vaccines is in the way, presented by the author, only speculation and not supported by any evidence based study. His speculation has been made only in very indirect way.
Concluding, I do not support publishing of the chapter'.

Reviewer 3 commented:

'This paper does not have any major strengths. It does not address a testable question in a scientific manner. It says crazy things, like genetic changes are driven by immunization. REJECT!

This paper is not based on science. It starts with the premise that vaccinated individuals have a higher incidence of autism than non vaccinated and the references that are used are not mainstream. This appears to be a paper that is not based on a true testable hypothesis as the data do not support the analysis that is performed. This paper should be rejected as it appears to be from concept to performance without merit. It appears to be non science'.

We reject these criticisms. We do not believe that this article is pro vaccine or anti-vaccine. It is hoped that the article is pro-science. We have further revised this article and place it in the public forum and now ask our readers to make their own conclusions.

Graham Ewing 8th November 2013

About the Author

Graham Ewing is Chief Executive of Montague Healthcare. He has devoted the period 2003 until the present to a programme of work which is designed to commercialise Virtual Scanning technology.

This technology is significant for a number of reasons. It is based upon a unique mathematical model of the autonomic nervous system which links cognitive input to cellular & molecular biology. This has immense diagnostic and therapeutic significance. It means that we can determine the onset of pathologies in terms of their influence upon the body's systems, organs, cells and ultimately in terms of phenotype and genotype of each pathology.

Virtual Scanning was developed by Dr Igor Gennadyevich Grakov during a program of research conducted at the University of Novosibirsk in the early 1980's which was intended to explore the medical application of industrial lasers. It was during this research that Dr Grakov established a biological response to a waveform i.e. to monochromatic light.

Graham Ewing has devoted much of his time to assembling a scientific explanation for this technology. As a result he has become the author of circa 50 peer-reviewed medical articles and conference presentations. He has also compiled a book and has been invited to compile several book chapters several of which have now been published following peer review. He is regularly invited to submit articles, to attend medical conferences, and to give presentations. He has become a Systems Biologist of growing international repute and (by virtue of his work to commercialise Virtual Scanning) an authority on the relationship between cognition, the autonomic nervous system, and the physiological systems i.e. how sense perception and sensory coordination influence, and are influenced by, the autonomic nervous system and physiological systems and how autonomic dysfunction leads to changes of cellular and molecular biology.

This program of articles illustrates a number of issues which cannot be explained by contemporary biomedicine e.g. how the brain regulates, and is regulated by, the visceral organs; why 90% of drugs are ineffective in 50% of patients; why most contemporary diagnostic tests can never be a precise measure of a medical condition; the significance of genotype and phenotype in pathologies; why complementary and alternative medical techniques and/or therapies can have a therapeutic effect and to what extent; why flashing lights can cause photosensitive events and why light and light-based biofeedback techniques can have a therapeutic effect; how an understanding of the autonomic nervous system could conceivably reduce the need for organ transplants; and what are the fundamental causes of migraine, developmental dyslexia and regressive autism.

This understanding of the autonomic nervous system has indicated how Virtual Scanning is based upon a principle which, in principle, may be more significant and advanced than any current diagnostic technology including biomarkers or genetic screening; how sensory input influences cellular & molecular biology; how it is able to determine the onset of pathologies, earlier, better (in terms of genotype and phenotype), more comprehensively (all systems and organs), safer (non-invasively), faster (results in circa 15 minutes), and at significantly lower cost than contemporary means of diagnosing the onset of pathologies (less than half the cost of current techniques); and how it is the first technology which could be used to determine the complete health of the vast majority of the world's population. It has also illustrated how the therapeutic application of light may have the potential to stimulate protein reactivity and hence improve therapeutic outcomes from circa 50% which is obtained by using drugs, to a level of typically 75-95% by using Virtual Scanning Light Therapy.

Printer

Printed by Lightning Source, Milton Keynes

Notice

Statements and Opinions expressed in this book are these of the author and not necessarily of the printer or publisher. No responsibility is accepted for the accuracy of the information contained in the published chapters. Readers are requested to check out the facts, to independently assess the validity of the arguments assembled by the author, and to make their own conclusions.

The author, printer and publisher assumes no responsibility for any damage or injury to persons or property arising out of the use of any methods, or ideas contained in this book.

ISBN

ISBN 978-0-9556213-1-4

Quotes

'One likes to think of science as divorced from personality because one seeks the guidance of a principle rather than a person. Thus the individual scientist experiences a feeling of freedom since he has the impression he lives in a community in which the law and not the man is the ultimate arbiter. This truly democratic process has led to the fallaciously democratic process of determining the validity of a scientific view by determining how many other scientists agree with it. Voting in this context is so much influenced by past training and indoctrination that it tends to reject the new and reaffirm the old'.

Carl Lindegren

"Great spirits have always encountered violent opposition from mediocre minds."

Albert Einstein

"If we knew what it was we were doing, it would not be called research, would it?"

Albert Einstein

Beware of trying to understand the whole by the arbitrary isolation of the separate components or by hazy or forced abstractions."

Albert Einstein

"It takes 50 years to get a wrong idea out of Medicine, and 100 years a right one into Medicine."

John Hughlings Jackson, FRS1878

'The scientific establishment is permeated with opinions which pass for valid scientific inductions and with contradictions which are disregarded because it is too painful to face the prospect of revisions of the theory which would be required to reconcile the contradictory observations with the dominant theory'.

Carl Lindegren

"All truth passes through three stages. First, it is ridiculed. Second, it is violently opposed. Third, it is accepted as being self-evident."

Arthur Schopenhauer

What Causes Regressive Autism? Could it be the genetic and epigenetic consequences of the overuse of vaccines, their influence upon the autonomic nervous system, and the subsequent elimination of Mercury and heavy metals?

Author: Ewing G.W.

Affiliation: Director, Montague Healthcare

Abstract:

The occurrence of Regressive Autism is a multi-systemic disorder which is attributable to genetic, epigenetic and chromosomal abnormalities. The unvaccinated do not appear to suffer from Regressive Autism and appear to be significantly less susceptible to a wide spectrum of disease. The evidence suggests that such genetic and epigenetic changes arises from the overuse of vaccines, which subsequently influence cellular & molecular biology, and hence alters the fundamental mechanism which regulate the body's function i.e. the autonomic nervous system and physiological systems. Cognitive dysfunction and, in particular, alterations to sense perception are associated with changes to the stability and function of the autonomic nervous system and the function of the physiological systems. Consequently it is possible to consider the significance of autistic symptoms from a systemic perspective. The progressive failure of the eliminatory systems influences the elimination of heavy metals and facilitates their accumulation and subsequent manifestation as neurotoxins: the long-term consequences of which would lead to neurodegeneration, and the cognitive and developmental problems which are typical of mercury poisoning.

This article explores the issues from a cognitive and systemic perspective. It concludes that sensory dysfunction and progressive systemic dysfunction and failure, manifest as a spectrum of autistic disorders including regressive autism, is the inevitable consequence arising from significant levels of genetic and epigenetic alterations arising from the overuse of vaccines.

Key words: Regressive Autism, physiological systems, autonomic nervous system

Abbreviations: ANS: Autonomic Nervous System, GWS: Gulf War Syndrome; MMR: measles-mumps-rubella vaccination; ASD: Autistic Spectrum Disorder; SIDS: Sudden Infant-Death Syndrome.

Table of Contents

1. Introduction
1.1 A Brief History of Autism

2. What Causes Autism?
2.1 No-one knows and No-one is to Blame
2.2 Autistic Traits
2.3 Sub-types of Autism

3. What is Autism?
3.1 The Systemic Nature of Physiology and Function
3.2 The Cerebellum
3.3 The Influence of Sensory Input
3.4 Contraction of the Visual Field
3.5 Evidence of Autonomic Dysfunction
3.6 Evidence of Systemic Dysfunction in Autism

4. Vaccines and Vaccine Side-Effects
4.1 Background
4.2 What are the risks from diseases against which a Vaccine is meant to protect?
4.3 What are the Risks from the Vaccine? Typical vaccine side-effects
4.4 Effectiveness of Vaccines/Vaccines are not 100% effective
4.5 The Effect of Viruses and Vaccines upon the Learning Process
4.6 The Unvaccinated
4.7 Single Vaccinations vs Multiple Vaccinations

5. Biochemical Evidence
5.1 Biochemical Instability
5.2 The Use of Drugs
5.3 The Cause of Regressive Autism
5.4 The Influence of Heavy Metals

6. The Influence of Viral-RNA and other Gene-altering Factors

7. Current Therapeutic Approaches to Treat Regressive Autism

8. Discussion

9. Conclusions

1. Introduction

1.1 A Brief History of Autism

The occurrence of Regressive Autism has risen steadily in the last decades. In the UK, before the introduction of vaccinations, autism was almost unknown. By 1968, when Polio and DPT vaccines were administered to children of 6 and 7 months, autism remained quite rare. Doctors often recommended a 3 month period between vaccines. By the late 1970's the occurrence of autism was estimated to be circa 3-5 per 10,000; the majority of such cases having occurred from birth (1). By the early 1980's evidence emerged of a perceived link between MMR vaccination and the increased occurrence of regressive autism (2). In 1988, when Polio and DPT was given at 3 months, DPT at 5 months and MMR at c13 months, autism rates were still low however by 1996 the rate had begun to rise rapidly. Polio and DPT/HIB injections were administered at 2, 3 and 4 months, followed by the MMR vaccine at c13 months. The onset of regressive autism rarely affects children before 12 months. The rate at which vaccines were being given had increased significantly. The uptake of the MMR vaccine increased and coincided with a significant increase in the occurrence of type 1 diabetes (3-5). The occurrence of autism increased 10 fold by 2006.

Since the introduction of the modern intensive vaccine schedule, including multiple vaccines, the prevalence of autism has increased to an estimated 1 in 88 i.e. 114 per 10,000; and the trend is for a continued increase. Some estimates are that severe Autistic Spectrum Disorders (ASD's) now affects one in every 88 children (6,18). This is supported by research which suggests that circa 1 in 100 British children may have some form of autism (7) and that ASDs are far more prevalent than hitherto imagined (8) i.e. only severe cases of autism are statistically noted. *It raises the spectre that ALL children, perhaps with the exception of unvaccinated children, are being affected to some major or minor degree i.e. affecting their health, behaviour and education.* Such claims have been dismissed as mere speculation because there is not yet definitive proof of such claims however the perceived lack of evidence does not indicate that proof does not exist (9,10). What is clear is that educational standards, and the ability of children to learn, are continuing to decline (11-13). What is also clear is that the numbers of children who develop Regressive Autism is at a level which is without precedent. The lack of an explanation indicates that the understanding of the condition remains 'beyond the prevailing level of knowledge' (14) or that the issues are so delicate that it is difficult for them to be openly discussed.

By 1985 the incidence of regressive autism was similar to that from birth and by 1997 both types of autism had increased although, by then, the regressive form was >75% of the total occurrence i.e. an acquired condition had become greater than the level of birth defects (15,16).

Regressive Autism occurs to a greater extent in immigrants and descendants of immigrants from Africa who have a greater racial predisposition to autism (17) e.g. in Somali's living in Minneapolis there was a rate of 1 in 28 which compares with the local average of 1 in 56 and the national rate of 1 in 150. Black Americans and Hispanics also have a significantly higher incidence of regressive autism than white Americans (18,70). Since the 1960's the number of vaccines given to a child before entering school is now more than 33. In children born to military families, who are subjected to greater levels of vaccination, the occurrence of autism may be as high as 1 in 67 which appears to indicate that excessive amounts of vaccinations creates chromosomal abnormalities. Autism affects four boys to every girl (19). By contrast regressive autism does not appear to occur in communities which do not use vaccines (20-23) or in unvaccinated children.

Table 1: Rate of Occurrence of Regressive Autism

Period	Occurrence	Ave	Reference
Before the 1930's	unknown		
By 1968	rare		
Before 1980	3-5 per 10,000	4	
By 1985	6-10 per 10,000	8	
By 1997	30-35 per 10,000	32.5	(15)
By 2001	60 per 10,000 (1 in 166)	60	(32)
By 2002	less than 1 in 100	100	
In 2009	no sign of plateauing		(16)
In 2012	1 in 88	114	(18)
Estimated 2025		225	

In the vast majority of cases, the emergence of autistic indications appears to happen in children who had developed normally (19,24,25), and before three years (26,27). The development of normal function appears to cease in the second year (28) which is coincident with the schedule of vaccines (29) and/or the MMR vaccine (30,31). The prevailing medical opinion is that this is an unexplained coincidence.

Graph 1: Rate of Occurrence of Regressive Autism

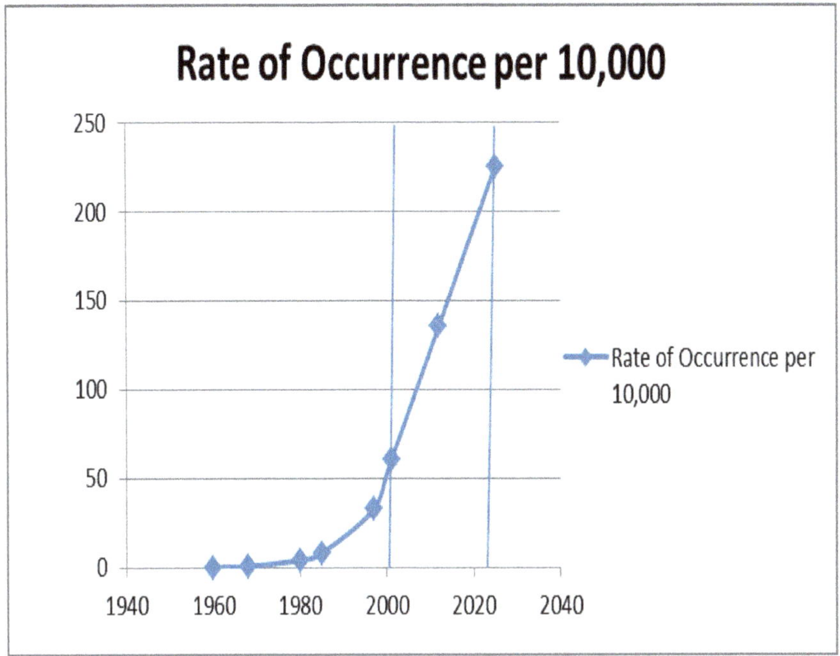

Rate of Occurrence of Regressive Autism (per 10,000) in the period 1960-2012 (including a projected estimate for year 2025).

Irrespective of the ultimate causative factors, the consequences to society are estimated at c£2.4M in an autistic child's lifetime (32) which, if it continues to increase as many predict, will impose an unsustainable financial burden upon healthcare, education (33) and social welfare systems throughout the world. It is therefore a political imperative for all in the world's population (not just in the UK) to address the issues, to understand why this condition occurs, to understand how to treat this condition and improve the lives of the many children which have been blighted by this condition, and to understand what can be done to prevent its future occurrence.

2. What Causes Regressive Autism?

2.1 No-one knows and No-one is to Blame

In common with most other medical conditions, Autistic Spectrum Disorders has genetic and epigenetic origins but it is also recognised that the environment plays a significant role in the etiology of ASD's. Arguably and controversially, especially so in the case of regressive autism, this has often been attributed to multiple vaccination, in particular the multiple MMR vaccine, however despite vehement denials by the medical profession the argument refuses to die. Parents with apparently healthy children prior to vaccination watch helplessly as their children develop autistic traits following vaccination (34,35) yet the medical profession fails to offer a viable explanation for this condition.

Whereas in almost every other medical consultation the observation and comments of the parent or patient is taken into account and used to determine an appropriate course of action, by contrast in the case of regressive autism and other autistic spectrum disorders their observations and opinions are often completely dismissed or ignored. Thereafter the parent has to fight for the resources to manage and raise their damaged children. 'Big Brother' is deemed to know best yet 'Big Brother' cannot offer the answer and insists that the MMR vaccine, or indeed any other vaccine or combinations of vaccines, does not cause regressive autism. Moreover that the experts cannot give a satisfactory and scientifically credible opinion is an issue worthy of further deliberations. The argument is not helped when noting that many conscientious researchers have lost their jobs when attempting to raise this issue i.e. of vaccine side-effects. The scientific debate continues in the manner of two pugilists slugging it out but without a clear winner or at least without one of the contestants being able to land a knock-out punch.

Scientific integrity and subterfuge have become so intertwined that they prevent anyone making a logical conclusion (36).

Some consider that the use of vaccines has become a belief system which is more powerful than the underlying science. The system of addressing the problem has become paralysed. No-one addresses the conflict of interest i.e. that someone who is part of the process of authorising the use of a vaccine would be compromised and would be biased against the withdrawal of the vaccine which they had recommended. No-one is held to be accountable for the increasing occurrence of regressive autism however independent legal rulings have accepted that, at least in some cases, vaccines have been responsible for the onset of regressive autism in some children. Nevertheless the prevailing medical opinion is that there is not a link between the use of the MMR vaccine and the occurrence of regressive autism. This may indicate that the cause is not solely with the MMR vaccine but instead with the wider principle i.e. that of multiple vaccinations and/or with the co-incident administration of single vaccines.

Regressive Autism can affect one of identical twins and has been linked to epigenetic changes (37). Children of medical doctors have developed regressive autism and other ASD's. Children of aristocratic families have developed regressive autism. No aspect of society is immune from this insidious insult however there are communities which have a greater susceptibility to such conditions e.g. the children of families of Somalian and Central African origins (18) who have chosen to live their lives in an environment which is not conducive to their health e.g. in northern Europe or the north-east United States. Such families have lower immune function due to the colder and light deprived environment by contrast to that which their skin requires to metabolise calcipotriol (vitamin D) and hence maintain a satisfactory level of immunity i.e. calcipotriol is essential to maintain a satisfactory level of immune function. In addition children who live downstream from coal-fired power stations have greater exposure to environmental Mercury and appear to be more vulnerable to autistic-type disorders (38). This indicates that there is a spectrum of genetic and non-genetic causes involved in the etiology of the condition.

There are a number of issues to consider e.g.

(i) unvaccinated children

In general, unvaccinated children do not develop regressive autism and other ASD's. This will be considered to be controversial i.e. it is considered to be unethical to withhold vaccination therefore the medical profession does not have control groups which can be used to test this claim. Nevertheless such data is held by groups which have a moral or religious exemption. The available information appears to indicate that unvaccinated people have significantly lower levels of illness and morbidities (20-23,39-42) i.e. that vaccinated children have significantly greater levels of diabetes, thyroid disease, migraines, epilepsy, scoliosis, autoimmune disorders, hyperactivity, hay fever, otitis media, herpes, sinusitis, asthma, bronchiectatic disease and allergies. Furthermore, the occurrence of regressive autism is less common in sparcely vaccinated communities (20-23).

(ii) modified vaccine schedule

Other countries/children of parents who select a modified vaccine schedule which involves fewer vaccines with greater gaps between vaccines appear to have less prevalence of ASD's e.g. the withdrawal of some vaccines (43,44) has reduced the incidence of disease whilst a delay or refusal to vaccinate has been associated with reduced risk of disease (45-47). The rate of infant deaths mirrors the numbers of vaccines. The more vaccines administered per child the greater the risk of death (48). See Table 2 and Graph 2.

(iii) whether other illnesses follow vaccination

The introduction of the MMR vaccine was followed by a steady increase in the occurrence of type 1 diabetes (3-5) i.e. that the genetic expression of pre-pro-insulin has been suppressed and that genetic or epigenetic change(s) have occurred. A similar effect was noted following the introduction of the BCG vaccine (49,50), haemophilus influenza B (HiB) (51,52), hepatitis B (53,54) and pertussis (55). In addition, further morbidities and mortalities occur following vaccination of adults e.g. in the US the adverse risk of mortality within 60 days of vaccination is circa 0.13% i.e. 13 in 10,000 (56).

Table 2:

Infant Mortality Rate/1000 births vs No of Vaccines Given before 1 year

Territory	IMR*	Vaccines Before 1year	Vaccine Schedule
Singapore	2.31	17	DTaP (3), Polio (3), HepB (3), BCG, Flu
Sweden	2.75	12	DTaP (2), Polio (2), Hib (2), Pneumo (2)
Japan	2.79	12	DTaP (3), Polio (2), BCG
Iceland	3.23	12	DTaP (2), Polio (2), Hib (2), MenC (2)
France	3.33	19	DTaP (3), Polio (3), Hib (3), Pneumo (2), HepB (2)
Finland	3.33	13	DTaP (2), Polio (2), Hib (2), Rota (3)
Norway	3.58	12	DTaP (2), Polio (2), Hib (2), Pneumo (2)
Czech rep	3.79	19	DTaP (3), Polio (3), Hib (3), HepB (3), BCG
Germany	3.99	18	DTaP (3), Polio (3), Hib (3), Pneumo (3)
Switzerland	4.18	18	DTaP (3), Polio (3), Hib (3), Pneumo (3)
Spain	4.21	20	DTaP (3), Polio (3), Hib (3), HepB (3), MenC (2)
Israel	4.22	18	DTaP (3), Polio (3), Hib (3), HepB (3)
Slovenia	4.25	15	DTaP (3), Polio (3), Hib (3)
South Korea	4.26	15-17	DTaP (3), Polio (3), HepB (3)
Denmark	4.34	12	DTaP (2), Polio (2), Hib (2), Pneumo (2)
Austria	4.42	23	DTaP (3), Polio (3), Hib (3), HepB (3), Pneumo (3), Rota (2)
Belgium	4.44	19	DTaP (3), Polio (3), Hib (3), HepB (3), Pneumo (2)
Luxemburg	4.56	21-23	DTaP (3), Polio (3), Hib (3), HepB (2), Pneumo (3), Rota (3)
Netherlands	4.73	24	DTaP (4), Polio (4), Hib (4), Pneumo (4)
Australia	4.75	24	DTaP (3), Polio (3), Hib (3), HepB (4), Pneumo (3), Rota (2)
Portugal	4.78	21	DTaP (3), Polio (3), Hib (3), HepB (3), MenC (2), BCG
UK	4.85	19	DTaP (3), Polio (3), Hib (3), Pneumo (2), MenC (2)
New Zealand	4.92	17	DTaP (3), Polio (3), Hib (2), HepB (3)
Canada	5.04	24	DTaP (3), Polio (3), Hib (3), HepB (3), Pneumo (3), MenC (2), Flu
Ireland	5.05	23	DTaP (3), Polio (3), Hib (3), HepB (3), Pneumo (2), MenC (2), BCG
Greece	5.15	23	DTaP (3), Polio (3), Hib (3), HepB (3), Pneumo (3), MenC (2)
Italy	5.51	18	DTaP (3), Polio (3), Hib (3), HepB (3)
Cuba	5.82	22	DTaP (3), Polio (3), Hib (3), HepB (4), MenBC (2), BCG
US	6.22	26	DTaP (3), Polio (3), Hib (3), HepB (3), Pneumo (3), Rota (3), Flu (2)

Graph 2: IMR vs Number of Vaccines administered before 1 year

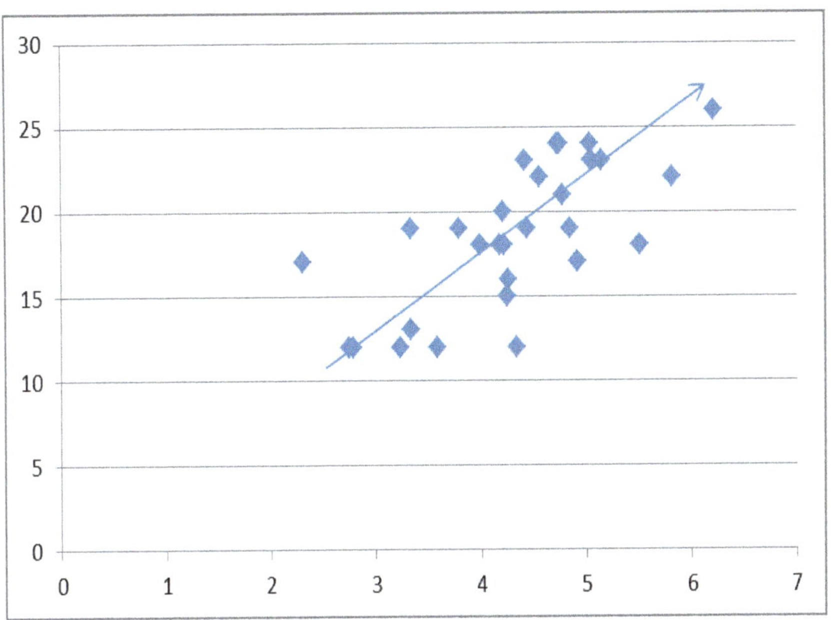

Infant Mortality Rate per 1000 Vaccinated Children

(iv) before and after vaccination

The occurrence of infectious diseases has changed with improved sanitation, better nutrition, and the modern vaccination schedule however many of the common viruses declined significantly, in some cases by 90-99%, before the modern vaccine schedule was introduced (57). Some diseases have declined naturally without any need for vaccination.

Despite the huge amount of scientific research there has not yet been a double-blind clinical study on any vaccine which compares the health of the vaccinateds with the unvaccinated over many years. If so, it cannot be possible to consider whether there could be benefits from withdrawing vaccines, adjusting vaccine schedules e.g.

(i) withdrawal of the smallpox vaccination in the 1980's led to a reduction in the incidence of tuberculosis;

(ii) the decline in the occurrence of scarlet fever in the 19th century was followed by lower incidence of measles and diphtheria;

(iii)Japan withdrew the MMR vaccine in 1993 because a record number of children had developed a wide range of adverse reactions and despite switching to another MMR vaccine in late 1991 the incidence of adverse effects remained high (57);

(iv)a study (58) claimed that there was no effect on the incidence of regressive autism when the MMR vaccine was withdrawn yet graphs in the report (59) clearly illustrate that rates of autism, dropped significantly in the following year i.e. as expected if the incidence of regressive autism in the 1-2 years age group was due to the combined effect of the MMR and other vaccines.

(v) how does the occurrence of Regressive Autism vary throughout the world

There is no recognised vaccine schedule which covers all countries. Different vaccine strains may be used in different countries. The numbers of vaccines administered varies from typically 10 - 30+ vaccines. Some countries use single vaccines whilst others have adopted multiple vaccines. In North America the rates of regressive autism vary between the populated centres where access to vaccination is easier and there is greater enforcement of the modern vaccination schedule (typically 65 per 10,000); and the Native American population which has a rural lifestyle (typically 23 per 10,000) and less rigorous enforcement of immunisation schedules. The susceptibility to regressive autism appears to increase with the amount of vaccines administered (60). It is reasonable, therefore, to consider that the overall vaccination burden or the co-incident administration of single vaccinations may be associated with the occurrence of regressive autism (61) i.e. the greater the number of

vaccinations the greater is the incidence of regressive autism (see Graph 2).
In addition, the occurrence of mild autistic traits such as developmental dyslexia tends to be greater in the most vaccinated countries. The occurrence of dyslexia is circa 5% in Japan which (Table 2) is one of the least vaccinated countries whilst the occurrence of dyslexia is circa 15-20% in the United States which is one of the most heavily vaccinated countries (367).

2.2 Autistic Traits

Autistic children exhibit traits which are often indicative of autonomic dysfunction, and of changes to sense perception and sensory coordination (62). It influences their perception of light, sound, touch, and perhaps also smell and taste. Their levels of sensory input are significantly impaired (see section 3.3). As the biochemical correlates of sensory input influences the autonomic nervous system (ANS) it follows that a decline in cognitive function is the inevitable consequence of emergent pathologies. Accordingly the perception and coordination of sensory input must also be affected in those with regressive autism (63,64) i.e. changes to the autonomic nervous system including the flow of metabolites influence brain function and the regulated function of the sensory and visceral organs. Changes at the cellular and molecular level i.e. of metabolites, influence brain function and vice versa.

It raises the possibility that we are seeing a spectrum of cognitive, physiological, and/or autistic disorders of greater or lesser degrees of severity (368) e.g.

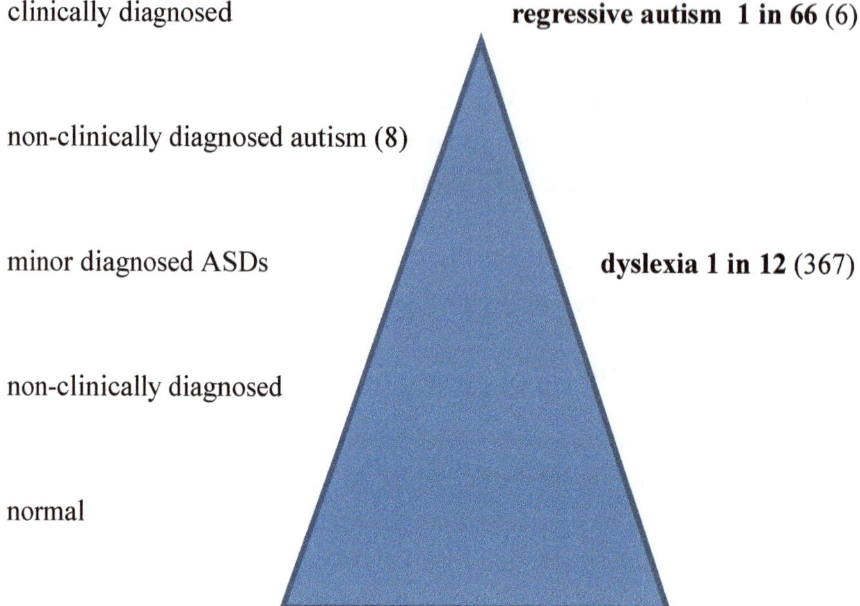

2.3 Sub-types of Autism

Autism is manifest in different levels of physiological and cognitive dysfunction e.g.

- Altered brain wave patterns in the autistic (65)
- Autism with problems of elimination e.g. of Mercury and heavy metals (66-68)
- Autism with epilepsy (69)
- Autism with gastro-intestinal disorders (70,71)
- Autism with temperature problems (111)
- Autism with sleep problems (72,73)
- Autism with cognitive/ sensory/behavioural problems (74-76)
- Autistic with abnormal blood pressure (77)

Autism is a problem of systemic dysfunction in which genetic and/or epigenetic changes influence systemic stability and function. The autistic brain is faced with the challenge of maintaining the body's stability when faced with a range of pathologies which collectively influence the neuro-regulation of the various physiological systems i.e. the emergent pathologies are of sufficient magnitude and complexity that the brain, in particular the pre-frontal cortex, is unable to maintain the body's regulated function. In some cases the dysfunction is associated with the instability of a single physiological system e.g. in some autistic children their autistic symptoms recede when they contract a viral infection which raises their body temperature. In others the evidence suggests that their autism is manifest as structural changes in the brain and the dysfunction of more than one physiological system. If it was due to a single vaccine we would likely see a precedent with a single virus but there are few allegations that a child has contracted autism following a single vaccination.

People rarely contract more than one virus at a time. This may be due to the generally raised levels of immunity in response to an infection. It may also explain why a child given a multiple vaccination or more than one vaccination coincidently or within a short period could be vulnerable to develop regressive autism i.e. that the body 's immune function responds to a single virus/vaccine which is compromised in those with a low level of immunity.

It is commonly considered that vaccines are designed to prevent the onset of a viral infection however Jenner's basic concept was not based upon preventing infection, but instead of giving an infection i.e. the cowpox virus acted to prevent infection by the more virulent smallpox.

The administration of a vaccine has been accompanied with increased virulence of other virusses e.g. pneumococcal vaccines have increased the prevalence of H.Influenza and of related upper respiratory tract infections (78); the chicken pox vaccine has increased the occurrence of shingles; the polio vaccine has significantly increased the rates of non-polio acute flaccid paralysis (NPAFP) (79,80); the H1N1 vaccine has increased the rate of occurrence of narcolepsy in vaccinated children (81); the DTP vaccination provoked an increase in polio (82); the MMR vaccination increased rate of measles encephalitis (SSPE) (83); etc. Viruses insert their RNA into DNA. Accordingly *the greater the influence of viral RNA the greater will be the potential to alter the structure and function of DNA.* This principle has been further recognised by the development of bacterial vaccines (84) which specifically seek to alter the structure of DNA and hence reduce the ability of viruses to infect.

This will have a positive or negative effect. Every single biological/genetic alteration influences genetic structure and the ability of the genes to express a protein (85). The recent ENCODE project has illustrated that many, many thousands of genes influence the body's regulated function. As genetic and epigenetic changes influence the expression of proteins including GPCR's, which link the body's internal and external interfaces, it follows that the greater the number of vaccines given in a short time-frame, co-administered, or given as multiple vaccines must increase the risk of visceral and sensory dysfunction.

The immune response organises the collective action of different immune chemicals e.g. immunoglobulins, t-cells, neutrophils, etc; in order to prevail against a particular virus. This mechanism requires the involvement of calcipotriol, and essential minerals. It must also be influenced by the prevailing intercellular pH and temperature. If so, how does the collective immune response deal with more than one virus (or similar/modified virus) at a time? Consider that the brain is a computational entity; continuously monitoring and adjusting the body's physiological stability (86,87). It faces an almost impossible task when dealing with the co-administration of many vaccines. *How does the brain, or for that matter the body, decide which of the vaccines administered in a multiple vaccination it should prioritise?* If faced with the co-administration of more than one vaccine how does the body manage to compute, discern or manage this process; in particular, where prevailing low levels of immunity is endemic e.g. due to lack of exposure to natural sunlight, lack of exercise, poor diet, inadequate consumption of calcipotriol in the diet, etc?

The use of vaccines depends upon there being a normal or satisfactory level of immune function i.e. that there is a sufficient level and spectrum of immunoglobulins, calcipotriol, t-cells, minerals, cofactors, etc; to perform the function of creating an antibody and hence of mitigating the onset of a viral infection. In many cases an adjuvant such as Aluminium is required to stimulate the immune response. This is recognition that the vaccine suppresses the prevailing level of immunity. If not, why have an adjuvant? This illustrates that a deficit of any single biochemical component is likely to compromise the immune response (88-90) i.e. in cases where a child has an impaired level of immunity, perhaps as a result of low levels of calcipotriol, the action of a vaccine will be less than expected.

"Have reason and logic abandoned epidemiologists?"

"The intentional, unnecessary introduction of infectious viruses into a human body is an error deriving from profound ignorance of virology and the process of infection. The ill that it does is incalculable".

Delong R. Live Viral Vaccine, Biological Pollution. pub Carlton Press, NY 1996)

If it is an inherited genetic problem why is this not a factor in those who have not been vaccinated? The evidence suggests that the coincident administration of many vaccines may have caused chromosomal damage. Clearly there are genetic and epigenetic changes which occur in response to viruses. *If so, the same phenomena must also apply to any products such as vaccines which adopt a similar principle i.e.* the use of vaccines must in some way alter our DNA. The immune response declines in the period following vaccination, often precipitating a susceptibility to viral infection, before recovering in the post vaccination period. The vaccination creates the memory of the immune response i.e. the ability to produce immunoglobulins; which the body uses to guard against future infections. It is our genes which are encoded to produce such proteins. This enables us to conclude that the issue is genetic. Vaccines influence our genetic profile.

A significant problem for virologists is that viruses are continually mutating and creating modified viruses against which a vaccine is increasingly ineffective. Moreover the recipient of the vaccine may previously have been vaccinated with many other vaccines. If so, the genetic profile must differ between patient groups. *Accordingly, and as stated earlier, the principle developed by Jenner no longer appears to be valid. Jenner's principle is based upon giving a viral infection (cowpox) to prevent an infection by smallpox. It is not based upon the principle of preventing infection.* It does not consider the genetic implications i.e. that reducing the vulnerability to one particular virus by immunisation could increase susceptibility to another virus yet any changes to the structure of DNA must inevitably change the susceptibility to other viruses. Vaccination is intended to prevent viral infection, at least to the specific virus, however evidence is accumulating that the extensive use of vaccines is creating a susceptibility to other infections e.g. (i) the flu vaccine leads to susceptibility to other flu variants, (ii) the use of polio vaccines leads to other polio variants, (iii) the use of malaria vaccines leads to the evolution of mutated and vaccine resistant variants, (iv) that some viruses can enhance immunity, and (v) that other diseases are becoming more prevalent.

The body rarely encounters more than one viral infection simultaneously. This happens because the immune response rapidly stimulates the levels of immunoglobulins and other biochemicals which are essential to maintain levels of immunity. When the body does encounter more than one viral infection the body appears unable to effectively deal with both viral contaminants e.g. (i) in a patient/sufferer of herpes simplex and other related viruses a mild seasonal influenza or cold can trigger an outburst of the sores and other symptoms which are a common feature of herpes type infections; (ii) infection by HIV makes the patient susceptible to other bacterial and viral infections which under normal circumstances i.e. in a patient who did not have HIV, would not cause anything more than mild discomfort.

A child born with little innate immunity is dependent upon the mother for the supply of mothers milk which provides the baby with immunity against a wide range of viral and bacterial pathogens (91). It is only after abt. 6 months that a child's natural immune function develops yet modern vaccination schedules do not take into account a child's level of development e.g. (i) of a pre-term baby (n.b. the advance in modern medicine allows a child to survive from as early as 20 weeks i.e. up to 18-19 weeks before their natural birthdate), (ii) whether the child is being breast-fed which will confer immunity for up to and beyond the first 6 months. Despite this the modern vaccine schedule requires that a child take its first vaccination from as early as 8-12 weeks after birth which may include children who have been born before its full-term birth date and before the innate immune response has developed fully.

3. What is Autism?

In order to explain what is Regressive Autism we must consider how the body regulates its function:

3.1 The Systemic Nature of Physiology and Function

The body is a bio-dynamic and systemic organism in which the brain regulates the body's function. It responds to sensory input which influences the ANS thereby influencing behaviour, the regulated function of the physiological systems and visceral organs (see figure 1). It also responds to biological input through the lungs, skin, digestive system, and the elimination of wastes and toxins. Changes to the levels of individual biochemicals, conceivably the consequence of changes to brain structure and function (62), influences the way that our organs function and hence how we act. This association between visual perception, the ANS, physiological systems, and cellular & molecular (63,64) raises issues which may be relevant to autism research e.g. the onset of pathologies influences colour perception (92,93) and the visual field; drugs alter colour perception (94); many proteins are visually active (95,96); suppressed immune function affects cognition (97) e.g. t-cell deficiency (a common indicator of stress) is linked to cognitive dysfunction. Such biochemical fluctuations influence sense perception and sensory coordination. The existence of the physiological systems is not in doubt although there is not universal agreement on their structure. They form the basis of a doctor's medical examination. There is wide recognition that they regulate the function of organs (in each system), and that there are higher and lower levels for each system (homeostatic limits), however such systems remain an elusive and under-researched area of medicine. The Russian researcher I.G.Grakov (98,99) has mathematically modelled the consequences of cognition upon the ANS and physiological systems.

Physiological Systems: Sleeping, Breathing, Digestion, Excretion, Osmotic Pressure, Blood Pressure, Blood Cell Content, Blood Volume, Blood Glucose**,** Sexual Function, pH, Temperature, Posture and Locomotion.

There is no recognition of an immune 'system' but instead that the immune function is provided by the co-ordinated function of all physiological systems and the function of the spleen, lungs, musculo-skeletal structures i.e. bone marrow, and gastro-intestinal tract.

Each system comprises a network of organs which work in a concerted and coherent manner. For example (i) the system with regulates pH comprises: Brain, Pituitary Gland, Thyroid Gland, Adrenal Gland, Liver, Pancreas, Lungs & Bronchi, Skin, Stomach, Duodenum, Kidneys, Large & Small Intestines, and Blood and Peripheral Blood Vessels; (ii) the system which regulates sleep comprises: Brain, Pituitary Gland, Spinal Cord, Peripheral Nervous System, Ear & Nose.

The brain waves appear to be in a dynamic relationship with molecular biochemistry. This may indicate how drugs can be used to influence the body's biochemistry in order to act upon the symptoms of disease and how brain wave technologies such as neurofeedback can be used to alter the brain waves, and the coordinated function of the physiological systems, organs, cells and molecular bio-chemistry. Such systems regulate the function of the body's biochemistry e.g. (1) most enzymatic reactions in the body are temperature dependent and catalysed by Magnesium and Zinc; (2) the body requires maintenance of pH within a narrow operating range, and also the supply of minerals and vitamins/cofactors, to catalyse protein-substrate reactions in the body; (3) appropriate blood volume, blood pressure, blood cell content, osmotic pressure and pH are required to ensure optimal absorption of minerals, vitamins, glucose and fatty acids from the intestines; (4) genotype and phenotype influence and are influenced by changes to sensory input i.e. genotype and phenotype alter colour perception.

The synchronised activity of groups of neurons (100) in functionally coherent structures (the physiological systems), which exist in the brain *and the body*, synchronise their electrical impulses (101). This may be evident when noting the evoked visual potentials, indicative of neural synchronisation, which are atypical in autism (102) and which may be part of the processes influencing sense perception (figure 1), sense coordination, memory (103), learning, etc. Sensory input is integrated into actions, behaviour and movement. In addition, learning requires synchronised activity between the brain, sensory organs (104-106), and visceral organs. This is severely disrupted in the autistic (107). Autism affects the function of all of the brain (108-110). It is a neurobiologic, multi-systemic disorder i.e. affecting the function of the brain and every organ but not necessarily its structures (111). It affects all aspects of the ANS and hence influences all aspects of brain's function including that of the neural networks which are involved in learning, memory, the function of the senses and the visceral organs.

Figure 1: Sensory Input, Neural and Visceral

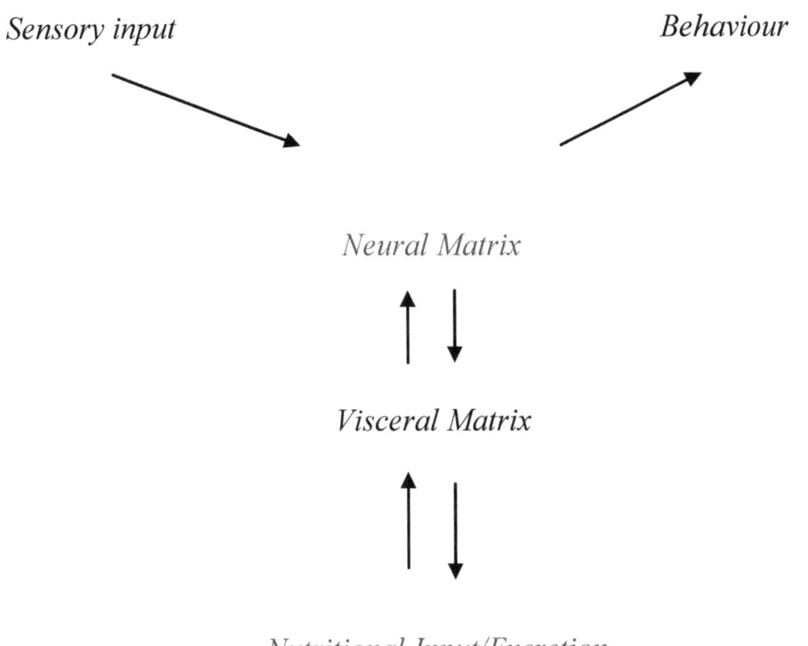

Every vaccination or drug depends upon the autonomic nervous system. They do not function independently of the autonomic nervous system. Accordingly it is the function of clinical studies to discern, if possible, the effect of the vaccine or drug in contrast to the body's innate healing mechanism.

3.2 The Cerebellum

The cerebellum, considered to be implicated in autistic spectrum disorders (112) comprises an estimated 50% of the brain's total processing capacity yet its role is not clear or understood (113). It is involved in the accumulation of sensory data from the internal environment, including the organs in the body and those in the brain (including the sensory organs), thus distinguishing between sensory input from the external environment (a significant function of the cerebrum) and that of the biochemistries affecting the function of every organ (a significant function of the cerebellum), including the cerebellum. Such a role includes the processing, regulation and distribution of this data, through structures such as the Purkinje cells in the cerebellum which are attached by nervous structures to every part of the body. It includes the receipt of biosignals involved in the processes of movement, coordination and balance. Reduced flow of data to the brain via the cerebellum (and brainstem) may lead to functional problems affecting the body's fine control of e.g. balance, coordination, etc. Movement and balance involve the coordinated function of all body systems and organs and are coordinated by (1) sensory feedback from the external and internal environments and (2) the allocation of energy resources to and from each organ. They are dependent upon the precise nature, and timing, of data about each organ being provided to and by the cerebrum *and* cerebellum. The brain determines behaviour and actions appropriate to developing situations. It illustrates how changes at the organ, cell or molecular level influence brain function and vice-versa. There are indications of cerebellar dysfunction in autism (114). Inhibited flow of data (see Section 3.3) to the cerebellum may be followed by developmental decay, cerebellar dysfunction (115,116), and reduced size of brain-stem. It is the equivalent of the 'use it or lose it' phenomena affecting muscle tone and function.

3.3 The Influence of Sensory Input

Without sensory input the brain cannot and does not function. Both disease and drugs alter sense perception, the visual field, and affects colour perception. In the case of Regressive Autism such changes are particularly evident. Moreover, such phenomena must have a biochemical basis. Alteration of sense perception, and in particular of colour perception, occur because proteins are visually active i.e. they emit bioluminescence. This emission of light influences our perception of colour. The colour and intensity of this bioluminescence is unique to specific pathologies and to the rate of reaction. Alterations to the level and nature of emitted proteins e.g.

as glycated proteins in the case of diabetes, influence the spectrum and intensity of this bioluminescence. Accordingly, changes to sense perception must have genetic, epigenetic and phenotypic significance. This is especially significant for the study of autistic spectrum disorders because vaccines are also associated with changes to sense perception.

Our cognitive function depends upon the extent and coordination of sense perception i.e. between the eyes, ears, nose, mouth and skin. The significance of an event arises from the coordination of sensory inputs. Genetic and/or environmental influences affect sense perception, the degree of sensory coordination and ultimately our awareness of our environment. Visual function is linked to the primary mechanism (rods, cones and pigments) but is also influenced at the biochemical level – noted by how emergent pathologies and drugs alter colour perception (117) and affect the neurovisual pathways which alter colour perception and visual contrast. This influences the stability and function of the ANS (118) and alters the processes of memory fixation, concentration, and behaviour (119).

3.4 Contraction of the Visual Field

The visual field of the autistic, determined by Syntonic Optometry, is influenced by their health. See figures 2-4.

Figure 2: **an Autistic patient**

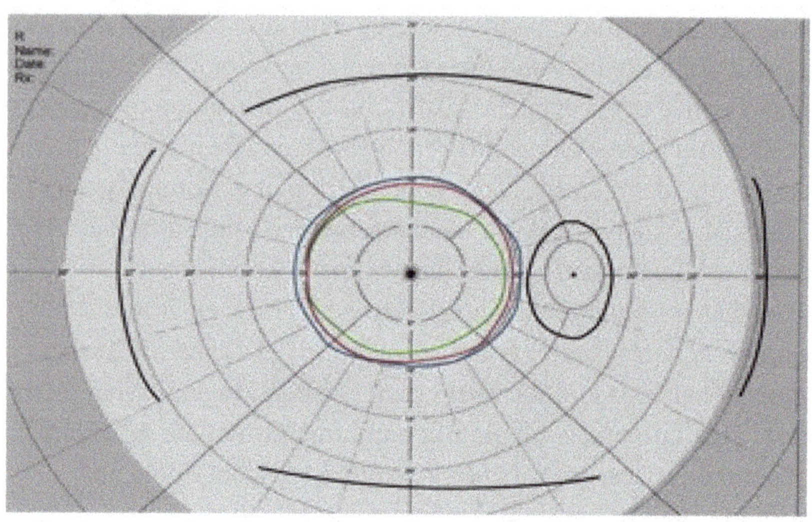

Figure 3: **a patient suffering from Depression**

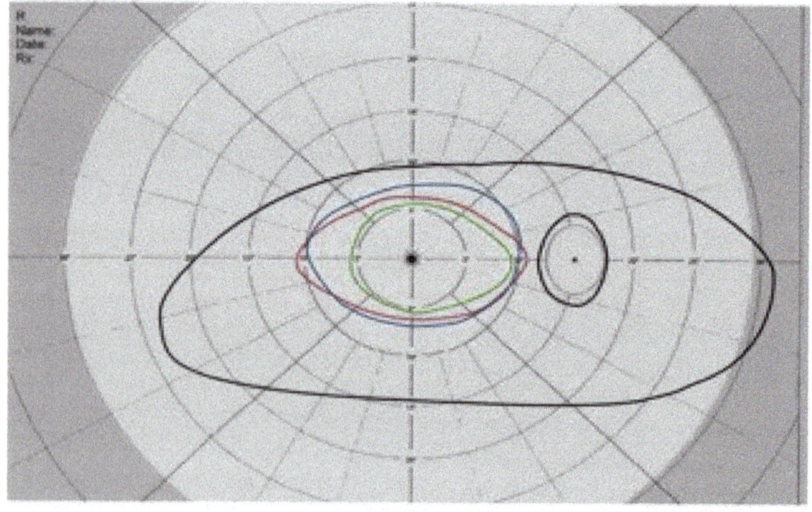

Figure 4: **Normal patient**

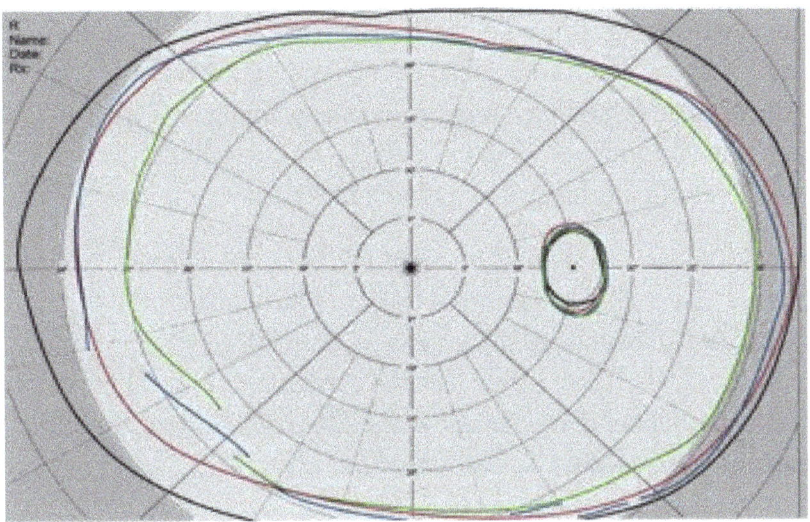

The large field (figure 4) is a 'normal' patient; the small field (figure 2) is of an autistic patient; and the other (figure 3) is a person who was emotionally traumatised, depressed and confused. The example autistic patient receives massively lower levels of visual input. The example depressed patient receives an estimated 20-30% of normal visual field/input by comparison to the normal patient. The origins of the depressed patient and the autistic may be different but the overall effect upon their visual field is clear. This lack of sensory input can be expected to influence to different extents their physical behaviour, balance, agility, and their ability to establish emotional relationships which require the exchange of sensory data.

Anyone contracting disease e.g. measles, mumps, rubella, tetanus, etc; experiences some alterations to visual perception therefore a weakened strain of the disease e.g. administered by vaccine, must also influence visual perception/cognition. This is a noted side-effect of many vaccines. Chronic disease is also accompanied by significant cognitive dysfunction and influences the coordination and processing of sense signals by the brain. The greater the number of illnesses, drugs or vaccines (120) the greater the alteration to the body's biochemistry therefore the greater its influence upon individual senses e.g. sense perception, sensory coordination, the degree of sensory distortion, speed of movement, memory, etc. It influences the ANS and physiological systems and hence the coordination and function of every organ – visceral and sensory - which is a significant feature of autism (121,122).

Almost all diseases are linked to cognitive and behavioural disorders. Conversely, behavioural traits are influenced by biochemistry e.g. testosterone, oestrogen, cortisol, oxytocin, adrenaline, etc. Oxytocin influences the formation of social bonds, social engagement and attachment - which are dysfunctional in the autistic child (123-127).

3.5 Evidence of Autonomic Dysfunction

As sense perception is linked to the stability of the autonomic nervous system and physiological systems (62,128) we would expect to see, in the autistic child: evidence of loss of sense perception and sensory coordination; system dysfunction (e.g. influencing breathing, blood pressure, blood cell content, heart rate, digestion, temperature, pH, osmotic pressure, sleep, etc); behavioural dysfunction (including learning problems, information feedback); problems with diet and elimination (of toxins and wastes); impaired and/or delayed neural development; atypical brain waves; etc. This is what we find in the autistic child/adult.

3.6 Evidence of Systemic Dysfunction in Autism

Autonomic dysfunction i.e. dysfunction of the autonomic nervous system and physiological systems, is commonly associated with a wide range of physiological disorders e.g. diabetes and obesity (129), cancer, cardiovascular disorders, pre-eclampsia, dyslexia (130), depression, sleep disorders, breathing disorders, etc. Changes to the stability of the central and autonomic nervous system are the hallmarks of autism in children (131). Systemic dysfunction in

Autism influences the regulation of temperature, blood cell content and immune function (132), blood pressure (133,134), digestion, excretion, posture and locomotion, sleep (135-137), pH, breathing; respiration rates, lower skin temperature. Each influences metabolic rate (138). Autonomic dysfunction has also been linked to problems with appetite, swallowing food, nausea, recurrent vomiting, and abdominal bloating; constipation or diarrhoea; dry eyes, dilated pupils; dry skin, flushed skin following a meal, abnormal sweating, and unexplained high fevers; sleep apnoea, insomnia; bed-wetting, difficulty urinating, difficulty potty-training; altered perception of pain, sensory defensiveness, poor socialisation skills, anxiety, phobias, tics, emotional instability; and light intolerance. That autistic seizures are often linked to neural blood flow (139-141) is supported by fact that medications used to raise or lower blood pressure alter the occurrence of seizures and improve sleep in the autistic child.

Autism affects sensory processing and sensory coordination (142) which is manifest in various ways e.g. tactile perception (143), vision (144), hearing (145), and smell. Autistic children may also display a form of synaesthesia i.e. sensations become confused with one another (146). Sounds may be experienced as touch or as visual stimulation e.g. autistic children may cover their eyes when they hear a loud sound. That autistic children have such sensory synaesthesia and sensitivity may indicate that their brains have extreme problems with sensory processing, regulation and coordination (147,148).

4. Vaccines and Vaccine Side-effects

Vaccines are considered by many to be the greatest advance in modern medicine (149) enabling the large-scale eradication of vaccine preventable diseases e.g. the worldwide eradication of smallpox; a massive decline in the incidence of polio; the prevention of hepatitis B infection and the subsequent development of cirrhosis, liver cancer and other complications.

The critics of vaccines point out that the current vaccine schedule is associated with a wide range of vaccine side-effects; that vaccines are not subject to double-blind clinical studies; and that the follow-up of the vaccinated rarely continues beyond several weeks i.e. before the development of vaccine-related side-effects.

By contrast the proponents of vaccines accredit the policy of vaccination with general improvements to world health e.g. the eradication of smallpox and minimising the occurrence of tetanus, measles, mumps, rubella, cervical cancer (Human Papilloma Virus); contributing to our increased longevity; and perhaps also contributing to improvements in women health, wellbeing and lifestyles.

The critics point out that the argument has been accepted but that it has never been proven beyond doubt; and moreover that all vaccines carry a risk e.g. of viruses mutating into more severe strains, which are drug resistant, and of vaccine-related side-effects.

4.1 Background

The proliferation of many viruses is seasonal. Their occurrence often rises during the autumn and winter (typically November to April) and declines during the spring i.e. when natural levels of immunity are at their lowest. Viral infections are rarely encountered during the summer months i.e. some viruses proliferate when the natural level of sunlight, and hence the antiviral effect of the UV in natural sunlight, is lowest; and when the body's immune function is at its lowest. The same effect is noted in the Southern hemisphere.

Measles often occurs, firstly and to a greater extent, in those parts of the country (S Wales, the Lake District) where there is greater levels of rainfall and consequently lower levels of exposure to natural sunlight. The statistics for the occurrence of disease and the administration of vaccines are readily available (www2.nphs.wales.nhs.uk).

The recent measles epidemic which occurred in South Wales in the UK started during the winter months of 2012. It was finally declared to be ended on 1st July 2013 following a long and severe winter yet an estimated 100,000 people had refused to be vaccinated. Moreover many in this epidemic contracted measles after they had been vaccinated with the MMR vaccine.

Indeed such considerations places in doubt the need for vaccination against measles if the child has adequate exposure to sufficient UV-light e.g. gained through outdoors activities.

By contrast the notified incidence of mumps has actually increased during the summer months. Whereas it was present at a level of circa 3 per million, during the summer months of 2013 the notified weekly incidence increased to a level of circa 10 per million per week during the peak summer months – ***following the intensive MMR vaccination programme given to prevent the occurrence of measles, mumps and rubella*** - before declining to what appears to be the base level of abt 3 per million.

In addition, the notified weekly incidence of whooping cough (pertussis) peaked during the November-January period at a level of circa 9 per million before declining to circa 1-2 per million during the summer months.

In addition there are three other issues which have had a very significant effect upon the ability of viruses to proliferate (i) there has been significant improvements in the quality of the water supply throughout the world; (ii) there has been an improvement of the living standards in many parts of the world; and (iii) there has been a significant improvement in the access to a nutritionally beneficial diet. Moreover, many of the common viruses were in decline before the introduction of vaccines. See Graphs 3, 4 & 5.

There are different approaches to the design of vaccines. Each is designed to stimulate the production of antibodies and thereby inhibit infection. The introduction of modified live viruses as vaccines enable the virus to attach its genetic material into the cell which replicates i.e. the host cell continues to function whilst producing the viral protein. Immunoglobulins are a group of immune antibodies which in isolation or in combination with other immunoglobulins, t-cells, neutrophils, etc; act to combat the presence of viruses in the body.

Graph 3: the incidence of child measles mortality in England and Wales during the pre-vaccination period 1850-1965 declined from over 1000 deaths per 100,000 of those under 15 years to circa 10 deaths per 100,000 per year (150)

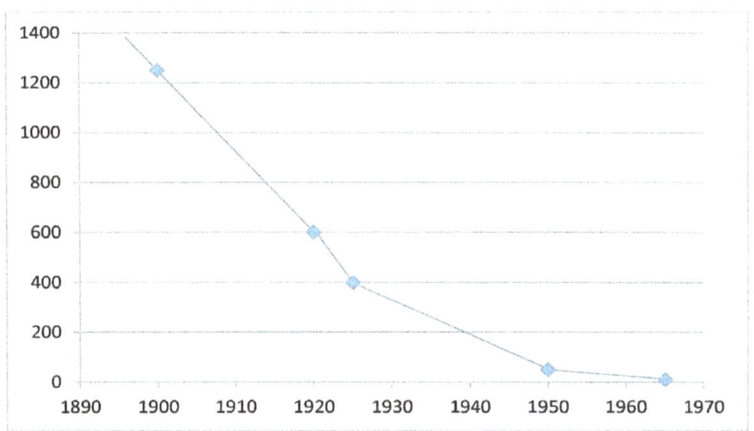

Infant Mortality Rate per 100,000

Graph 4: the incidence of child mortality in England and Wales due to measles during the period 1919-1967 was similar to that of child deaths due to scurvy (151)

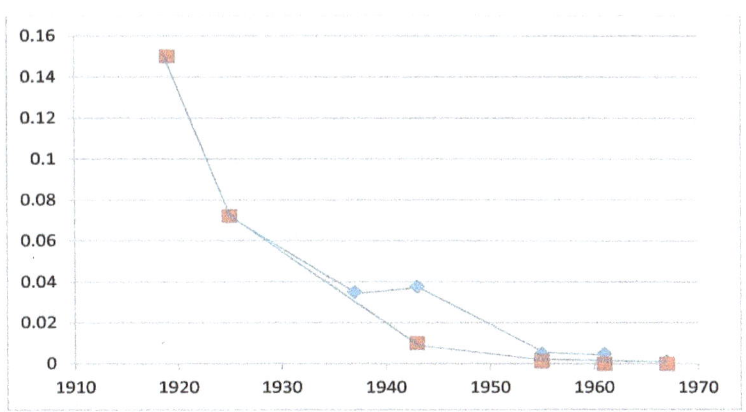

Incidence of Child Mortality

Note 1: Blue represents the incidence of scurvy whilst Red represents the incidence of measles. Note the blip in the graph due to the onset of WWII.

Graph 5: the incidence of deaths due to scarlet fever during the period 1910-1958 declined from over 12 deaths per 100,000 per year to zero without any need for vaccination (152)

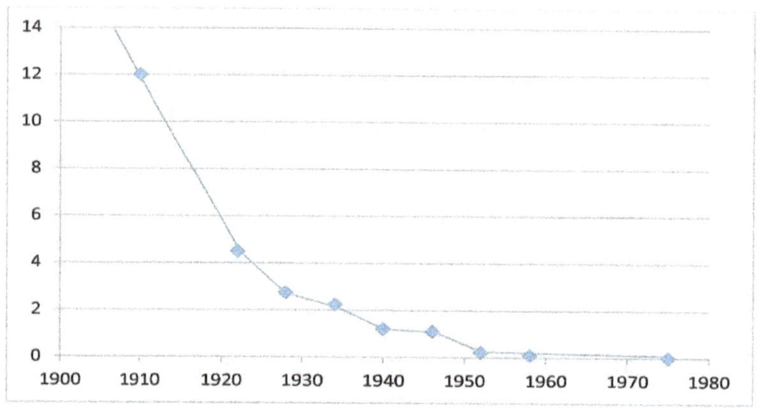

Deaths due to Scarlet Fever during the period 1900-1975

Under normal circumstances exposure to a viral disease would be countered (in vivo) at various levels enabling the body to steadily increase its immune response. By contrast, the injection of vaccines directly into the blood system by-passes or overpowers the normal immune response leading to its rapid depletion. It prevents the body's immune function from responding at the point of infection and hence of steadily upgrading its response as the infection progresses. It is suspected that long-term persistence of viruses and other proteins may produce chronic disease i.e. instead of producing a genuine immunity the vaccines are altering the body's systemic and biochemical stability, suppressing the production of differing types of white blood cells and hence the prevailing level of immunity. Furthermore the introduction of many vaccines (up to 30 in a typical vaccination schedule) introduces a large number of foreign proteins which may be sufficient to ensure that immune function never returns to baseline and/or that immune biochemistry is fundamentally altered. Consequently there now exists a growing concern which links immunisations to the huge increase in recent decades of auto-immune diseases (153) e.g., rheumatoid arthritis (154,155), multiple sclerosis, lupus erythematosus, lymphoma, leukemia, autoimmune demyelinative optic neuritis, diabetes mellitus, etc.

Vaccinations influence the balance of viral scavengers (156,157). They suppress the production of b-cells, t-cells, etc; which indicates that they are influencing, temporarily or permanently, the genetic expression of these key proteins. The synergistic action of these cells impairs antibody formation and becomes less effective in phagocytosis i.e. the mechanism which the body uses to remove bacteria, cell debris, etc. This influences recognition of viral pathogens, leads to the progressive failure of immune function and hence to the increased incidence of auto-immune disease which we note as allergies (158-160), immunodeficiency (161), etc. Some vaccinations have a greater effect than others e.g. Hib vaccine, pertussis vaccine (162-164), measles vaccine (165), etc. Indeed some articles indicate that the use of some vaccines can reliably induce asthma (166) by moderating adrenergic function (167).

All vaccines and viruses must alter the structure and function of DNA to some extent. It is inconceivable that it could have such effect unless it influenced genetic expression. Each virus is a large molecule therefore its spatial arrangement must influence the biochemistry affecting cross-helical structures and linkages within the DNA helix. The insertion of viral mRNA alters the structural conformation of DNA, and hence the expression of proteins. It is therefore inevitable that the steady accumulation of such foreign proteins arising from an intensive vaccine programme will reach the stage where it significantly weakens gene and chromosome structure and function. In addition, the prevailing reaction conditions which are the consequence of protein expression, and which have been influenced by previous vaccines, will also affect the introduction of each new virus. Each will depress immune function. The greater the number of viruses, vaccines and foreign proteins (1) the greater will be their influence upon immune function and the time required for recovery from each vaccination; (2) the greater their influence upon genetic, epigenetic and chromosome structure, the greater will be the effect upon protein function, system function/dysfunction, etc.

The greater the amount of vaccines, introduction of foreign proteins and hence of alterations to the body's biochemistry the greater the risk that the body's immune function no longer recognises or responds to existing vaccines or viruses (168) and/or that its immune response has been altered (169) e.g. sugar chains attached to an antibody alters its ability to bind to its receptors (170). This may lead to mutated forms of disease (171-178) e.g. the re-emergence of whooping cough (179), and a differentiated disease profile e.g. up to 30 per cent of individuals with a persistent cough are infected with B. pertussis (180). Furthermore enhanced susceptibility to viral infection as a consequence of vaccination are documented (181) and could enable tougher strains to flourish (182).

Most children are breast-fed. The mother's milk provides the baby with a level of immunity and hence of protection against many of the common infections yet the current vaccine schedule advises vaccination at 3-6 months irrespective of individual variation e.g. including premature birth. Accordingly it is suspected that vaccines may be administered prematurely. For example, giving the DTP vaccine to babies at 2, 3 and 4 months is considered to be less effective than giving the vaccine to babies of 3, 5 and 9 months i.e. they are less effective during the period when pertussis is most hazardous to a child's health.

Vaccines are not entirely safe (183). *If they were entirely safe governments would not have been required to provide indemnity against future claims by parents of damaged children.* The currently used vaccines are merely less unsafe than previous vaccines (184,185) e.g.

(i) the Urabe strain of mumps used in the MMR vaccine was replaced by the Jeryl Lynn mumps strain following reports from Japan of high levels of meningoencephalitis;
(ii) the Pluserix and Immramax-MMR vaccines were withdrawn because of reports of mild transient meningitis;
(iii) the Rubini vaccine remains in use despite safety concerns (186);
(iv) the Leningrad-Zagreb strain may have superior efficacy and is often used in developing countries (187,88);
(v) different strains of disease have different safety profiles (189);
(vi) different strengths of vaccine (190) carry risks which have a differing effect upon age groups and gender;
(vii) there are concerns over the use of whole-cell vaccines (191,192) and that acellular vaccines may be less effective (193);
(viii) the incidence of Sudden Infant Death Syndrome (SIDS) has been linked to the DPT vaccine (194) although in some countries the incidence of SIDS has been largely eradicated following withdrawal of the pertussis vaccine in Sweden and Japan;
(ix) vaccine side-effects include the onset of autoimmune disease (153,195) e.g. arthritis, type 1 diabetes, etc;
(x) sensory defects are a common side-effect of vaccines (196-198) e.g. hearing loss induced by the MMR vaccine;
(xi) some drugs may inhibit the effectiveness of vaccines (see 4.3.2) e.g. steroids suppress the immune system and increase the risk of infection from live virus vaccines (199);
(xii) vaccines may also be influenced by levels of immune function, diet, and stress (200);
(xiii) the occurrence of some diseases may have increased since the introduction of a vaccine (201).

> “If we look at the experience of the USA, the overall incidence of acute hepatitis B since vaccination for it began has not diminished but has increased from 55 to 63 per 100000 between 1981 and 1987. This disappointing result is not, however, unexpected: coverage of high-risks groups remains unsatisfactory”.
>
> Sicot C. Medico-Surgical Consultations. Le Concours Médical, No 8, 1993 (Vol 115)

Many, many parents of autistic children and a number of medical experts believe the MMR vaccine is the culprit behind autism. In circa 15-20% of children it causes fever shortly after immunisation yet the significance of this effect is largely disregarded.

4.2 What are the risks from diseases against which a Vaccine is meant to protect?

Diphtheria (202) is an upper respiratory tract infection characterized by sore throat and minor fever. It affects the central and peripheral nervous systems leading to deterioration of myelin sheaths, loss of motor control and sensation. Fatality rates are 5-10% although the rate of mortality may be higher for those under 5 years and over 40 years. It can be treated by antibiotics which prevent its transmission. Other minor complications including neck swelling, nausea, vomiting, listlessness, pallor, and a racing heart beat; lead to long term effects e.g. low blood pressure, cardiac myopathy and peripheral neuropathy. **Poliomyelitis** is an infectious viral disease which has been eradicated in the developed world as a result of improved sanitation. Although c90% of polio infections are symptom-free, if the virus enters blood circulation this may lead to further complications. In c1% of cases, where the virus enters the central nervous system, it infects and/or destroys motor neurons thereby leading to muscle weakness and paralysis, usually involving the legs. (There are now mutated forms of polio (NVAPF/PVAP) which are be responsible for polio-like disease in vaccinated children and adults (79) i.e. the efforts to eradicate polio by vaccination are causing the emergence of a polio-like disease). Some populations have developed immunity to the wild polio virus (203). **Tetanus** infection occurs through open wounds. It occurs mainly in hot, damp climates with soil rich in organic matter from ruminants. It creates muscle spasms in the jaw, difficulty in swallowing, muscle stiffness and spasms throughout the body. There are c1M cases reported each year, mainly in the developing world, causing an estimated 300-500,000 deaths. In the US, there are about 1-5 deaths from tetanus each year. It is the only disease that is infectious but not contagious. **Pertussis** is a highly contagious disease. There are 10–90 million cases and about 600,000 deaths each year. Sixty percent of all cases occur in the developing world. In children it is characterized initially by mild respiratory infection symptoms before developing into the characteristic 'whooping' cough. It is dangerous in babies which are particularly at risk. Complications include encephalitis, pneumonia, and secondary bacterial infections. **Hib** (H. influenzae) appears only to occur in humans with low natural immunity (204). In infants and young children, H. influenzae type b may cause pneumonia, and acute bacterial meningitis. Both H. influenzae and S. pneumoniae both reside naturally in the upper respiratory tract. Alterations in the immune response; attributed to poor nutrition, stress or transmission; facilitate their proliferation. **Measles** is largely the consequence of compromised immunity arising from poor diet and is linked to high levels of mortality (205) in the developing world (circa 28% although the rate of mortality from measles in the developed world ranges from zero to 0.3% e.g. there have been few, if any, recorded deaths from measles virus in the UK for almost 20 years. The classical symptoms of measles are typically fever (up to 40C), cough, coryza and conjunctivitis. Complications include mild diarrhoea, pneumonia, encephalitis, SSPC, and corneal ulceration or scarring. They are usually more severe amongst adults. Permanent hearing loss or damage to vision are recognised complications of measles. Measles has been known to occur in children with congenital rubella syndrome, and has been implicated in the etiology of inflammatory bowel diseases (IBDs). The more common symptoms of **Mumps** are parotitis, fever (typically 38.3C), headache and orchitis (206). Other symptoms of mumps includes sore face and/or ears, and loss of voice. Known complications of mumps include infection of other organ systems, sterility in older men, mild forms of meningitis, encephalitis, sensorineural hearing loss, pancreatitis, inflammation of the ovaries, and risk of spontaneous abortion during pregancy. **Rubella** is relatively benign and often passes unnoticed (207). The primary reason for the introduction of a vaccine is to prevent infection of mothers during pregnancy. The main symptom is a rash which appears on the face, trunk and limbs (after an incubation period of 14-21 days) which usually fades after several days. Other symptoms include fever (typically 38C), swollen glands (post cervical lymphadenopathy), joint pains, headache and conjunctivitis. Children exposed to rubella in the womb may show developmental delay, inhibited growth, hearning disabilities, diabetes, glaucoma, schizophrenia, etc. If infected during the first 12 week period of pregnancy this may lead to congenital rubella syndrome (CRS), which is manifest as a series of complications including spontaneous abortion and, in the neonate: cardiac, cerebral, ophthalmic and auditory side-effects. Known complications include prematurity, low birth weight, and neonatal thrombocytopenia, anaemia and hepatitis. CRS is the main reason a vaccine for rubella was developed. CRS is manifest as sensorineural deafness, eye problems, heart disease. Other complications include low birth weight, mental retardation, problems with the spleen, liver and bone marrow, etc. Mumps and Rubella may occur without the patient being aware that they have the disease e.g.c40% of mumps occurs in people who are unaware that they have this condition. Some diseases may confer natural immunity e.g. the mumps virus may confer a degree of immunity against ovarian cancer (208-211) therefore reducing the natural degree of exposure to mumps may increase susceptibility to ovarian cancer. Hepatitis B is difficult to catch and comes from blood or sexual contact with an infected carrier. Further, vaccine-derived immunity is thought to be short-lived. Hpv, an infection transmitted during sexual intercourse, clears naturally after several months/years. **Varicella** (Chicken Pox) is caused by the varicella-zoster virus. It is highly contagious. It begins with a mild fever, and a rash of red pimples which form itchy sores and scabs. It usually affects children of 1-14 years. It can be more severe in young babies, adults or people with an impaired immune system e.g. in adults it can cause shingles.

4.3 What are the risks from the Vaccine? Typical vaccine side-effects

There is evidence that BCG and measles vaccinations, when administered singly, reduce child mortality (212) but this is unrelated to the incidence of measles or measles deaths (213,214). By contrast the pertussis vaccine is associated with a negative effect (215). Side-effects of vaccines are indicative of systemic instability affecting most physiological systems – temperature (chills and fever), excretion (inflammation of the lymph glands), blood cell content (low platelet count), excretion (diarrhoea), digestion (poor appetite, vomiting), sleep (coma), and metabolic rate (tiredness, lowered levels of consciousness). In addition there is evidence of altered sense perception, indicative of problems with the autonomic nervous system, which affects hearing, visual perception (abhorrence of bright lights), smell and touch. For example (i) **DtaP vaccine** include *fever*, tiredness, poor appetite, vomiting and inflammation. Less common and more severe side-effects include distress (crying), seizures, lowered consciousness or coma, brain damage. (ii) Side-effects with the **MMR vaccine** include *fever*, swelling of the lymph glands, tiredness, poor appetite, and abhorrence of bright lights. More severe problems include low platelet count, pain and stiffness in the joints/ inflammation. Less common and more severe side-effects include distress (crying), seizures, deafness, lowered consciousness or coma, brain damage. (iii) Side-effects with the **Tdap vaccine** include pain, chills, *fever*, headache, tiredness, poor appetite, stomach ache, vomiting, diarrhoea and inflammation. Significant vaccine side-effects have been linked to swine flu vaccine (Guillain-Barre paralysis); in RSV vaccine (216); in the measles, mumps and MMR vaccines (217); hepatitis A and B vaccine (218); tetanus vaccine; smallpox vaccine; polio vaccine (NVAPF/PVASP); pertussis vaccine (219), influenza vaccine (narcolepsy/Pandemrix vaccine) (220); etc.

In developed countries, most children are immunized against measles by the age of 18 months, generally as part of the triple vaccine treating measles, mumps and rubella (children younger than 18 months usually retain measles antibodies (immunoglobulins (Ig)) transmitted from the mother during pregnancy). The MMR vaccine in particular has been linked to autism (221), Crohn's disease, inflammatory bowel disease (222,223) and other serious chronic stomach problems (224), epilepsy, brain damage including meningitis (225,226), cerebral palsy, pancreatitis (227) and diabetes mellitus (3,228,229), encephalopathy, encephalitis (230,231), hearing and vision problems, arthritis, behavioural and learning problems, chronic fatigue syndrome, diabetes, Guillain-Barre syndrome, idiopathic thrombocytopaenic purpura, subacute sclerosing panencephalitis (SSPE), leukaemia, multiple sclerosis, and death.

There is evidence that in cases of immune deficiency that viruses may continue to persist in the body (232-234). The measles virus is known to persist in patients with subacute sclerosing panencephalitis (SSPE), measles inclusion body encephalitis (MIBE) (235) and multiple sclerosis (236). Since the introduction of measles vaccine(s), vaccine-associated SSPE has increased in the USA. Furthermore patients with B or T-cell immunodeficiencies have cognitive side-effects (97) and are advised against vaccination due to the risk of severe and/or fatal infection (Merck). How does anyone know whether a child has B or T-cell immunodeficiencies at the point of vaccination? That viruses persist in the body and are linked to autoimmune disorders is also a feature of rubella virus (237-239), anthrax vaccination (240), hepatitis B (241), etc. There is a reported increased risk of death with combined vaccination DPT and polio (159).

In Nigeria the rate of deaths from Diphtheria *increased* significantly following the introduction of a vaccination programme in 1979 (242).

4.3.1 The Cumulative Effect of Vaccines

There is concern that the cumulative effect of vaccines upon the body's function has not been properly assessed (162). A multiple vaccination is not considered to carry any greater level of risk than any of the single vaccines, yet in pharmaceutical research, drug combinations have to be extensively tested and monitored to ensure their safety. It is *assumed* that multiple vaccinations are safe.

Unvaccinated children appear to have less exposure to disease (20-23,39-42), a less severe level of infection (34), delaying vaccination reduces exposure to disease (243), contracting the disease naturally leads to less disease in future (244), the virulence of future infections may be lower than if the disease was contracted by a vaccinated child (34), and that excessive vaccination is considered ineffective and dangerous (245).

The greater the number of vaccines administered - the greater is the rate of mortality in the under 5's (57). There does not appear to be available any international statistics for the rate of occurrence of regressive autism throughout the world which is surprising for a condition of such prevalence. Nevertheless the incidence of regressive autism appears to be greatest in the most heavily vaccinated populations e.g. Japan, US, UK; and is significantly less prevalent in the less vaccinated countries. In addition, it would be surprising of the relationship between the number of vaccines administered and rate of mortality in the under 5's was not accompanied by a similar increase in the rate of morbidities in the under 5's e.g. of conditions such as type 1 diabetes, regressive autism, etc.

4.3.2 Vaccine-vaccine and Vaccine-drug interactions

In general, vaccines may be influenced by antibiotics (246), immunoglobulins, immunosuppressants, monoclonal antibodies, anticoagulants and corticosteroids. The interaction between a vaccine and a drug has been reported only with influenza vaccine and four drugs (aminopyrine, phenytoin sodium, theophylline, and warfarin sodium), and with BCG vaccine and theophylline. The clinical significance of vaccine-drug interactions is not fully determined (247). There is evidence of interactions involving most vaccines e.g. HPV vaccine; shingles vaccine; yellow fever vaccine; polio vaccine (neomycin, streptomycin, phenoxy ethanol, formaldehyde), rotavirus vaccine, etc.

Vaccines are not subject to double blind clinical trials despite the evidence of vaccine-drug interactions and perhaps also of vaccine-vaccine interactions.

4.4 Effectiveness of Vaccines/Vaccines are not 100% effective

Pertussis is becoming increasingly prevalent (248-250). Although claimed to be 88 per cent effective among children of 7-18 months, during a nationwide epidemic of pertussis in 1993, a group of researchers discovered that 82 per cent had completed their full course of DPT vaccines (251) and in a recent outbreak in California in 2010 the majority of those who tested positive for pertussis had been vaccinated. Further outbreaks followed in Wisconsin, Washington and Vermont. B.Pertussis is suspected of being a factor in persistent coughs (179,180).The pertussis vaccine may be as little as 36% effective (184).

Many studies show that the measles vaccine isn't completely effective (252-255) and that a significant proportion of those infected in measles outbreaks (>60%) had been vaccinated. In 1985, in an outbreak of measles in Texas, 99% of those infected had been vaccinated (256); in 1993, in an outbreak of Pertussis in Ohio, 90% of those infected had been vaccinated (257); in an outbreak of Chickenpox in Oregon in 2004, 86% of those infected had been vaccinated (258); and in an outbreak of mumps in Iowa in 2006, 92% of those infected had been vaccinated (259).

There is also a lack of concensus concerning the effectiveness of whole or acellular vaccines, each having their own side-effects and effectiveness (260) e.g. vaccine efficacy was estimated at 75.4% for an acellular 5 component vaccine, 42.4% for an acellular two component vaccine and 28% for a whole cell DTP vaccine (261). The whole-cell vaccine was associated with different levels of side-effects in children including significantly higher rates of crying, cyanosis, fever, and local reactions; than the other vaccines. In the case of pertussis, there was concerns over the use of a whole-cell vaccine and an acellular vaccine was introduced to replace the whole-cell vaccine.

There is evidence of declining vaccine immunity (262) illustrated by transmission of mumps (263), measles (264,265), rubella (266), polio (267), Hib (268,269), Hepatitis B (270), smallpox, diphtheria, varicella (271), pertussis (272), influenza (273), etc.

4.5 The Effect of Viruses and Vaccines upon the Learning Process

One in 14 children in the UK i.e. up to half of all children starting school, have problems with speech, language, hearing (12) and communication (274). Is this significant bearing in mind (8) that the occurrence of autism and ASD's may be more widely spread than has hitherto been considered possible i.e. that only the most severe and chronic cases of autism are recorded? Learning problems are a significant problem in autism (275). It affects the body's processing of data from the external and internal environments. This affects the autistic's ability to make sense of the external world and the ability of their autonomic nervous system to regulate organ function and is part of a spectrum of biochemical disorders (77) which influence all aspects of the learning process e.g. including memory, concentration, sense perception and sense coordination.

4.6 The unvaccinated

Perhaps the most significant argument against the extensive use of vaccines comes from surveys which compare the vaccinated with the unvaccinated. Bear in mind that regressive autism was not prevalent in any communities before vaccines were introduced. There are three congregations from which this information can be drawn (i) religious exemptions i.e. populations which have a religious objection to the use of vaccination; (ii) parents who are concerned and who have withheld their child from vaccination; (iii) indigenous populations which have not been subjected to vaccination. The Amish (20-23) have a religious objection to the use of vaccines and have been surveyed and there is no evidence of any unvaccinated Amish having been diagnosed with regressive autism. In comparisons of vaccinated vs unvaccinated the vaccinated children are vulnerable to regressive autism as outlined in the introduction whilst regressive autism appears not to occur in unvaccinated children. In addition, they appear to experience a significantly higher level of disease, mainly in the form of allergies (39-42). So what causes an allergic response?

4.7 Single vaccinations vs multiple vaccinations

In the case of measles vaccination the Urabe 9 strain of measles does not cause any significant side effects when it is administered as a single vaccine yet when given in the MMR vaccination has been associated with the occurrence of vaccine side-effects.

5. Biochemical Evidence

So far this review looks at the effect of vaccines and diseases from a systemic perspective. It should also not be overlooked that drugs and vaccines depend upon the autonomic nervous system for their effectiveness. They do not and cannot work independently of the autonomic nervous system. Accordingly, it must be difficult to distinguish whether the effectiveness of a vaccine was due to the vaccine or the body's innate immune response. If so, it is essential to conduct studies which determine the effect of each factor.

5.1 Biochemical Instability

The health of a child with regressive autism is influenced by an astonishingly wide range of biochemical deficiencies e.g. (a) fatty acid deficiency (276); (b) a distinctly different immune response (79) incl. reduced natural killer cell activity (277); decreased levels of immunoglobulins; decreased levels of T cells; altered lymphocyte functions (278-281); and (c) vitamin D deficiency (282). Vitamin D regulates the levels of glutathione which may explain the link between heavy metals and autism. Depleted levels of glutathione facilitate increased levels of oxidative stress, suppress the detoxifying effect of liver enzymes e.g. P450, reduce the elimination of heavy metals, and increase the neurodegenerative effects of heavy metals. Mercury inhibits the enzyme methionine synthase which converts homocysteine into methionine. Accordingly, levels of cysteine, glutathione and metallothionine are low. This illustrates that the methionine pathway may be faulty in many with autism and supports earlier suggestions that redox imbalances (283,284) and detoxification are impaired. In addition vitamin D enables t-cells to function as viral scavengers. Other noted deficiencies include: (d) vitamin A deficiency (285,286); (e) carnitine deficiency (287); (f) increased norepinephrine levels and decreased dopamine-hydroxylase activity (288); (g) differences in serotonin binding sites by the antibodies from an autistic child (289); (h) altered levels of gut flora (290); (i) enterocolitis (291); (j) adenosine deaminase activity decreased in autism (292,293); (k) small intestinal enteropathy with epithelial, IgG and complement deposition in children with regressive autism (294); (l) mitochondrial disorder (295); and (m) that mitochondrial dysfunction, including abnormal enzyme function, mitochondrial structure, and mitochondrial DNA integrity, may be present in children with autism (296).

5.2 The Use of Drugs

As outlined biochemical instability is a feature of autism. Accordingly, drugs are often used to mitigate the autistic symptoms e.g. (i) Lofexidine (297) has been shown to stimulate prefrontal cortical function in nonhuman primates. This is consistent with the view that the prefrontal cortex regulates executive/system function; (ii) Methylphenidate may ameliorate hyperactivity (298), and impulsivity in autistic children; (iii) Neuroleptics e.g. haloperidol, are mildly effective in reducing hyperactivity, impulsivity, and inattention in children with autistic disorder (299); clonidine is used in the treatment of tic disorders and ADHD (300). Other drugs used in the treatment of autism include Tianeptine (301); Galanthamine (302); immunoglobulins (303); melatonin (304); and beta-blockers (305).

5.3 The Cause of Regressive Autism

It is now widely recognised that the occurrence of regressive autism is the consequence of a significant genetic or epigenetic insult (306,307) although it is not generally considered to be an inheritable condition. How and when this occurs can be debated however, for a young child with a developing immune system, there are few factors which could be held responsible other than vaccines and/or the related and damaging effect of exposure to high levels of Mercury and/or other heavy metals. No other explanation has been offered as a viable alternative explanation for the occurrence of regressive autism. A number of observations have been advanced e.g. altered brain connectivity (308), that males with regressive autism have larger brains (309), etc; but no-one has advanced any reasons to explain why these would occur.

- Over 100 genes have been identified which have been linked to regressive autism (307). Significantly, this includes some with X-linked chromosomal alterations.
- Genetic variants e.g. CNTNAP2 and MET are associated with risk of autism and altered brain connectivity (308).
- males with regressive autism have brains that are six percent larger than anyone with early-onset autism. The brains of females with regressive autism do not appear to show any difference in brain size (309).
- a link between regression and a family history of autoimmune thyroid disease, an association with gastrointestinal symptoms, etc.

The establishment including the most eminent of organisations e.g. the American Academy of Pediatrics and Institute of Medicine (2004) maintains that there is no link between vaccination and regressive autism (310) yet there is no common agreement on what is regressive autism and there is no concensus about what causes regressive autism. In fact there is no causal explanation, other than that of vaccination, which has been advanced by anyone. Moreover, that it occurs throughout the world and mostly in vaccinateds indicates that vaccination must be seriously considered as the ultimate cause of this condition.

If it looks like Mercury poisoning there is a very good chance that it is mercury poisoning. Thimerosal was used to preserve contact lens solutions but was withdrawn because of the toxicity associated with mercury-based preservatives. Around the world, Mercury is no longer recommended for use in mercury-amalgam tooth fillings because of the known toxicity of the mercury. In the UK and EC mercury can no longer be used in thermometers to measure temperature or in sphygmomanometers to measure blood pressure. See Note 2. So why is it permitted in any vaccines?

Note 2.

http://ec.europa.eu/health/ph_risk/committees/04_scenihr/docs/scenihr_o_016.pdf

http://ec.europa.eu/health/ph_risk/committees/04_scher/docs/scher_o_089.pdf

The evidence indicates there is alteration to chromosome structure and/or function. This is consistent with Mercury poisoning. It indicates the influence of external stressor(s) influencing mitochondrial structure and DNA (311), chromosomal instability and translocation, which ultimately influences protein expression. The combined effect influences system stability, organ function, the prevailing levels of biochemistry, sense perception, behaviour, etc. It influences protein expression and the rate and completeness of subsequent protein-substrate reactions leading to lowered immune function, reduced absorption of nutrients, slowed metabolism, impaired neural development (312) i.e. the body's biochemical processes do not proceed as they should and structural anomalies develop in the autistic brain.

Viruses are able to infiltrate cells by inserting their genetic material into them. Indeed Jenner's principle, based upon the observation that milkmaids contracted cowpox which made them immune to smallpox, is based upon the fact that the cowpox altered DNA.

As outlined earlier (see 4.1) there are biochemical markers of vaccine damage. That it affects four boys to every girl illustrates that the condition is largely due to a defect with the X-chromosome and leads to consideration of the factors which could influence at the genetic/chromosomal level. In general, chromosomal damage is linked to radiation e.g. due to adverse nuclear events which leads ultimately to birth defects. The prevailing evidence appears to suggest the influence of e.g. proteolytic enzymes or temperature (313,314) which may alter chromosome structure. Little evidence has been offered for the 1 in 5 occurrence experienced by girls although this also appears likely to be the consequence of a chromosomal stressor.

It is widely recognised that genetic predisposition and protein expression can be influenced by environment influences and that genetic damage can be the result of exposure to radiation, however the evidence being offered appears to suggest a subtle form of genetic alteration - associated with the wider use of vaccines - which may not necessarily be inherited but is responsible for altered system stability and function and consequently of altered biochemistry and function. There is evidence that, at least in some cases, system function may be intact but dysfunctional i.e. that homeostasis is severely compromised. This is indicative of epigenetic and/or genetic changes.

Research into Gulf-War Syndrome (GWS) identified (315) untypical RNA in the blood of sick GW veterans. It indicated that the viral encephalopathies originated from RNA-viruses and hence from vaccines. That immuno-suppression, shown to be a factor in GWS (316) and autism, is associated with the concentrated use of vaccines (317) is further supported by the fact that French soldiers who were not excessively vaccinated yet who served in the Gulf War did not get GWS; however American and British soldiers (318), irrespective of whether they served in the gulf war or not, reported a significantly greater incidence of autistic-spectrum disorders and GWS.

5.4 The influence of Heavy Metals

Heavy metals play a role in the etiology of a wide range of diseases (319) including, but not limited to, neurological disorders and autoimmune diseases (321). They act as catalysts in the oxidation of biological materials, induce reactive oxygen species (320), generate free radicals, etc. Consequently epigenetic alterations have been linked to the presence of heavy metals. Furthermore Mercury and Aluminium, often used as preservatives and/or adjuvants in vaccines, have been linked to epigenetic changes (322-325).

Heavy metals, and Mercury in particular, affect the function of the CNS. Their function has been extensively researched and associated with autism (326). Amongst a variety of side-effects mercury decreases lymphocyte viability, and in the brain: dysfunction in the amygdala, hippocampus, basal ganglia, and cerebral cortex; destruction of neurons in the cerebellum; and brainstem abnormalities which could reasonably be expected to lead to neural and systemic dysfunction. Demyelination is evident in such conditions. The brain's electrical patterns are similarly abnormal. The influence of mercury upon brain function cannot therefore be ignored.

In addition the body has an innate ability to eliminate toxins via the lymphatic system. It is necessary to consider why the majority of vaccinated children are able to eliminate Mercury and Aluminium from their systems whilst others who go on to develop regressive autism appear less able to eliminate such heavy metals.

The most significant contributors to the increased mercury load are: Mercury in vaccines (e.g. DTP (at typically 25 micrograms of Mercury/thimerosal per dose), Tetanus, Hepatitis B & (most) influenza vaccines), contamination of fish (327), wild/bush fires; dental amalgam; and emissions from power stations (328) and industrial chimneys including incinerators, waste-burning cement works, crematoria, etc. The characteristics of regressive autism and Mercury poisoning are extremely similar which suggests that it arises from mercury poisoning (329,330). This is supported by the observation that autistic children have greater amounts of mercury and other heavy metals in their systems (331). Vaccinated children of circa 10-20 kgs are exposed to an adult overdose of Mercury, over 62.5 micrograms of Mercury within the first three months, which significantly increases a child's risk of developing some form of neuro-developmental disorder such as impaired development, speech and language, autism, stuttering and attention deficit disorder. In addition, children living downstream of coal-fired power stations have a greater incidence of autistic spectrum disorders (332). This indicates that the innate physiological processes which the body uses to eliminate heavy metals are being overcome by overexposure.

Mercury poisoning is an insidious process. In general the symptoms do not appear immediately upon exposure. The initial preclinical stage is followed by the development of symptoms over a period which may last from weeks, months, and years (333-335). Consequently, Mercury given in vaccines to very young children would not be expected to lead to a recognizable disorder, except for subtle signs, before age 6-12 months, and might not emerge for several years (304). In autistic children, the initial signs occur shortly after the first injections, and consist of abnormalities in motor behaviour and in the sensory systems, particularly touch sensitivity, vision, and numbness in the mouth (336). These signs are followed by parental reports of speech and hearing abnormalities appearing before the child's second birthday (19). Finally, there is the development of autistic-like traits and a continuing regression or lack of development in subsequent years. These symptoms change (337) depending upon the circumstances surrounding each child. Most autistic children have impaired liver detoxification. In addition to the deficiencies outlined earlier, many have low levels of metallothionine, conceivably the consequence of a deficiency of Zinc, which is indicative of a lowered capacity to chelate Mercury and other heavy metals. Mercury is a powerful oxidant which depletes cellular antioxidants, especially glutathione. The P450 detoxifying enzymes of the liver rely heavily on adequate availability of glutathione. Ethyl Mercury the active component in thimerosal causes apoptosis of the t-cells (338-340).

Although the withdrawal of Mercury from some vaccines has not resulted in an overall decline in the occurrence of autism this does not mean that the problem does not lie with thimerosal (341,342). It may indicate that the problem is associated with the elimination of heavy metals incl. Mercury (342) e.g. an inflammatory response influences the lymphatic system which subsequently influences the elimination of neurotoxins (343). This is supported by noting evidence of urea cycle dysfunction. Problems with the urea cycle, conceivably the consequence of mercury poisoning, have been linked to autism. A child with ornithine transcarbamylase (OTC) deficiency is likely to be lacking in energy, have appetite problems, poorly-controlled breathing rate and/or body temperature, and slow development. Significantly, OTC deficiency is an X-linked recessive disorder (344) one of a number of primary immunodeficiencies associated with vaccine use. Other genetic/chromosomal abnormalities associated with regressive autism include: Phosphoribosylpyrophosphate (PRPP) synthetase superactivity, Adenylosuccinate lyase deficiency, Histidinemia, Lesch-Nyhan disease, Fragile X syndrome, Rett Syndrome, Dihydropyrimidine dehydrogenase (DPD) deficiency, Tuberous sclerosis, Superactivity of pyrimidine 5'-nucleotidase (P5N), etc. Genetic changes are associated inherited birth defects therefore it is reasonable to conclude that genetic changes must also be responsible for regressive autism.

As in autism, the onset of Mercury toxicity symptoms is gradual in some cases, sudden in others (266,267). In the case of poisoning, the first signs to emerge are abnormal sensation and motor disturbances. As exposure increases, these signs are followed by speech problems, and hearing deficits (345). Upon removal of the mercury the symptoms tend to recede except in instances of severe poisoning, which may lead to death (266). As in autism, epilepsy arising from Mercury exposure is also associated with a poor prognosis (346). Mercury acts upon the catecholamines and influences the function of the ANS (344). This affects cognitive performance (347), spatial vision (348), etc.

Other metals have been implicated in adverse neurodevelopmental outcomes in children e.g. lead and Mercury (349,350), with exposure to Aluminium, Cadmium, Arsenic, Copper, Antimony and Chromium also a concern. Studies have found adverse effects of prenatal Lead exposure on growth and development, but little research has examined an association with autism. Whilst Mercury is of concern, because of evidence for neurotoxic effects and the fact that it has become so prevalent in the wider environment (349), Aluminum also shares common mechanisms with Mercury e.g. it interferes with cellular and metabolic processes in the nervous system. Children given the recommended vaccinations are injected with nearly 5 mg of Aluminum by the time they are just 1.5 years old i.e. almost 6 times the safe level. Furthermore the nature of the Aluminium affects the prevailing blood levels and is also increasingly implicated in autism (351), through their use as vaccine adjuvants.

Nevertheless, despite the evidence outlined above, the connection between exposure to Mercury and vaccination has not yet been accepted. Mercury has been withdrawn from some vaccines as a precautionary measure but has been retained in many other vaccines. A recent study (352) adds to the evidence that Mercury influences neural function.

6. The influence of Viral-RNA and other Gene-altering Factors

Viral-RNA is a huge molecule. It inserts itself into our genetic structure. In doing so it alters the spatial and structural arrangement or conformation of our DNA. The energetic properties of the gene(s) are altered, the spatial orientation of each gene in relation to other genes is disrupted, and consequently the collective ability of the genes to express a protein are altered. In some cases e.g. type 1 diabetes, this results in a significant reduction of the ability to express a protein e.g. pre-pro-insulin and hence the levels of insulin.

Consider the implications e.g. a single nucleotide or sugar molecule can alter the virulence of a virus or the ability of an antibody to bind to its receptors (170). This means that the expression of an encoded protein(s) will be reduced but also that in some cases the ability to express an encoded protein may be enhanced. This would explain why some viruses appear to enhance the expression of encoded proteins and hence improve the prevailing level of immunity. It may also explain why some viral infections become entrenched e.g.

- up to 30 per cent of individuals with a persistent cough are infected with B. pertussis (180).
- some have an enhanced susceptibility to viral infection as a consequence of vaccination (181).
- some are infected with measles which is same strain as the measles vaccine.
- why bacterial vaccines (84) have been designed i.e. to alter our DNA.
- why viruses are now being considered to treat diabetes i.e. to partially reverse the recognised genetic changes.

Heavy metals are large molecules which adhere to our DNA/genes. This has an epigenetic effect which, like viruses, has an effect upon the structural conformation of our DNA. They have the effect of attracting electrons and hence of reducing the energetics of the DNA molecule. This has a number of effects e.g. (i) it alters the ability of the molecule to flex and/or rotate, (ii) influences the flow of substrates to and from the genetically active sites, (iii) prevents the flow of proteins and substrates to genetically reactive sites, (iv) alters the reactivity of the reactive sites which express proteins, (v) alters the replication of DNA, and (vi) leads to the expression of mutated proteins, (vii) may catalyse changes to DNA, etc. Accordingly the sequence of addition of each piece of viral RNA would be significant e.g. if DNA was introduced from three different sources in different order e.g. a-b-c, a-c-b, b-c-a, b-a-c, c-b-a, c-a-b; this would not lead to the same structural conformation and hence could result in different physiological outcomes.

The reduced level of protein expression e.g. of proteins which participate in the immune function, could enable hitherto benign proteins to become more virulent (179), may lead to mutated forms of disease (171-178), and would facilitate the emergence of new and tougher strains (182).

7. Current Therapeutic Approaches used to Treat Autism

There is little evidence that autism is a treatable disease although some therapies appear able to mitigate the effects of autism (353,354,363). Although there is no recognised method of treatment, or of significant and/or proven outcomes, autistic children appear to respond to therapies which enhance the function of the *breathing,* enhance oxygen levels (355), and the function of the *excretory* system e.g. by osteopathy (356). Moreover an occasionally observed side-effect with some autistic children is that when experiencing an elevated *temperature*, perhaps resulting from a fever, the autistic symptoms appear to recede and the child behaves normally (111). Autistic children suffer from adverse *sleep* patterns. In the US autistic children are occasionally treated by chelation therapy and neurofeedback (354,357-360). Dysfunction of the Excretory or lymphatic system leads to long-term exposure to Mercury which under normal circumstances would have been rapidly eliminated from the body. This may also lead to higher neural temperatures which will inevitably influence brain function.

There is evidence of biochemical deficits (360) and of the benefit of biochemical supplements e.g. vitamin B_6 and magnesium; melatonin; methylcobalamin; vitamin A, C & D supplements; dimethylglycine (DMG) and trimethylglycine (TMG). DMG provides building blocks that are required for purine nucleotide synthesis. DMG comes from TMG when TMG methylates homocysteine. Significantly, absorption of Vitamin A Palmitate requires an intact gut mucosa at the appropriate pH and in the presence of bile for metabolism. Many autistic children have damaged mucosal surfaces which impairs their capacity to absorb vitamin A (361).

That some children can become normal when their temperature increases above normal levels e.g. due to a viral infection (111), may illustrate that the levels of the homeostatic mechanism affecting the physiological systems have been reset at what can be considered to be abnormal levels i.e. that genetic and epigenetic changes are altering the fundamental levels of homeostasis. In addition, light can be used in neurofeedback therapies. Light influences the proliferation of viruses. In particular the UV component of natural sunlight stimulates the production of calcipotriol and calcitriol in the skin, which enable t-cells to function as viral scavengers.

In the absence of any approved therapies to treat Regressive Autism chelation therapies (354) have been used with some success, it is claimed, to reduce the levels of heavy metals increases in the Autistic. The technique is considered to be dangerous and has been associated with several fatalities due to e.g. hypocalcaemia.

In addition, alterations to the levels of digestive bacteria will influence brain function (see Figure 1). There are indications that autistic children have low levels of prevotella and several other species (362) indicating that the levels to the microenvironment which is able to sustain the function of these bacteria e.g. alterations to pH; levels of minerals, vitamins and cofactors; and proteins and substrates. Accordingly any efforts to rebalance the digestive flora can reasonably be expected to have some effect (363).

Other treatments being researched include the use of oxytocin, stem cells, and the developmental psychology technique ESDM.

8. Discussion

The evidence suggests that the onset of regressive autism may be linked with the modern vaccination schedule. The greater the number of vaccines which are administered the greater is the number of vaccine-related deaths and the number affected with Regressive Autism. No other reason has been offered which matches the facts. Denial is not a valid scientific methodology. Regressive Autism was not in evidence before vaccines, and/or when fewer vaccines were administered, and hence when there was a greater time between vaccines. Every virus, and hence every vaccine, which introduces viral RNA and/or otherwise evades the natural immune mechanism, influences the genetic profile and genetic conformation. This influences the spectrum of proteins which are genetically expressed and which in the autistic child has been severely affected. At some point the accumulated genetic and epigenetic variants and their influence upon our function will start to become evident. The mass of scientific evidence compiled by medical researchers indicates that the incidence of regressive autism increases following vaccination and is most closely associated with the intense schedule of vaccines including the MMR vaccine i.e. it occurs between year 1 and year 2 of a child's life. It occurs in children who have developed normally and who show no signs of dysfunction however, to date, there have been no studies which conclusively prove the link between the MMR vaccine and Regressive Autism (although they do not exonerate the MMR vaccine) i.e. the MMR vaccine may not be the cause of regressive autism but it may be a very significant contributory factor.

Following the measles outbreak in South Wales, the health authorities in England and Wales have used this opportunity to dramatically increase the uptake of the MMR vaccine. The current statistics (stated by BBC on 27th September 2013) is of circa 90% uptake by children of up to 3 years. This presents an opportunity to evaluate whether there is an increased incidence of Regressive

Autism and other Autistic Spectrum Disorders. If the incidence of Regressive Autism in South Wales increases in future, and in particular within the next 1-2 years, then the focus of attention will come to rest upon the use of vaccines.

Medical research accepts that genetic and/or epigenetic changes influence the expression of proteins yet the prevailing medical opinion is that this does not matter in the cases of vaccines! This ignores that the vaccine industry moved away from the use of whole cell vaccines, which contained foreign proteins, because of safety concerns i.e. the foreign proteins were responsible for causing high fevers. That vaccines suppress natural immune function is not in dispute e.g. those with low levels of immune function show greater predisposition to autistic spectrum disorders. Those who have a lower than normal immune function are recommended in vaccine guidance notes to avoid being vaccinated. This supports the view that the genetic spectrum is altered by vaccines.

The injection of a vaccine by-passes the normal multi-level mechanism in which the virus is identified and attacked by the body's immune function. A vaccine influences the genetic expression of proteins and hence of white blood cells including e.g. lymphocytes, immunoglobulins, t-cells, b-cells and/or neutrophils. It alters their synergistic action and hence their ability to memorise and respond to viruses when challenged. The immune response becomes compromised. The effect of the genetic and/or epigenetic insult to the neural mechanisms regulating system function affecting influences e.g. pH, the digestive and excretory systems, and the elimination of toxins and heavy metals i.e. mercury and other metals are retained instead of being eliminated. This may explain why the discontinuation of thimerosal in vaccines was followed by a steady increase in the incidence of autism and hence that researchers have not hitherto established a correlation between the incidence of autism and the use of thimerosal-containing vaccines. Irrespective, studies continue to demonstrate that mercury has an epigenetic effect which influences neural function (321).

It is not scientific to ignore that vaccines can cause genetic or epigenetic changes because viruses, bacteria and all manner of environmental influences including food and drink each alter our genetic profile to some extent. Gene therapies are being pioneered to correct a wide range of errors in the genetic code. It is therefore inconceivable that vaccines do not in some way influence gene function or that the mercury and aluminium from vaccines does not bind to DNA.

It offers a plausible explanation for the effect of multiple vaccines and concurrent administration of single vaccines and the greater predisposition to autistic spectrum disorders in military families. It offers a plausible explanation for those with darker skins, living in northern latitudes who have lower than needed levels of natural sunlight (particularly during the winter months) and hence have lower levels of calcipotriol, who appear particularly susceptible to regressive autism. Calcipotriol is necessary to the immune function of t-cells. Without adequate levels of calcipotriol immune function becomes significantly less effective.

Further support for the hypothesis that vaccines influence our DNA and hence the expression of proteins comes from the observation that sense perception is linked to the autonomic nervous system and physiological systems, and ultimately to cellular and molecular biochemistry i.e. genotype and phenotype. Alterations to sense perception and sensory coordination are indicative of genetic alterations and are features of autistic spectrum disorders (63). This is supported by noting how sense-based neurofeedback-type treatments are used with some effect to treat the mildly autistic (339) and the more severely affected autistics (74).

In most autistic children brain structures are initially unaffected but become steadily under-developed as a consequence of exposure to Mercury and other heavy metals e.g. there are significantly higher levels of Mercury in samples of hair taken from children with regressive autism. The brain of male autistic children becomes enlarged. The condition bears a striking resemblance to Mercury poisoning which suggests that Mercury, and perhaps also Aluminium, poisoning could be a precursor to a neurodevelopmental problem which leads to the development of chromosomal abnormalities, influences the degree of myelination, the onset of encephalitis, the function of the prefrontal cortex, the subsequent degeneration of the cerebellum, etc. If so the earlier that the autistic child can have Mercury or other heavy metals removed from their system can be expected to influence the rate and extent of recovery from regressive autism.

Regressive Autism can be manifest in many different ways. It exhibits the characteristics of an almost total failure of the body's regulatory mechanism which affects the autonomic nervous system, the stability of the various physiological systems, cellular and molecular biology, and the function and coordination of the senses. Occasionally it exhibits the characteristics of a syndrome which affects just one system. The accumulation of Mercury and other metals appears to indicate the progressive failure of the systems which eliminate such neurotoxins i.e. the lymphatic system.

The reduction of the visual field (see figure 2) illustrates how the flow of sensory input has been massively reduced to the autistic brain.

There is clearly an association between the numbers of vaccines administered and the rate of occurrence of Regressive Autism. If vaccines are administered coincidently or in a multiple vaccination how does the brain identify which should be prioritised? (A similar situation with the supply of data to a computer would result in the computer programme 'crashing'. Furthermore there is increasing recognition that biological systems have an innate ability to compute their response to an environmental event). As outlined earlier the immune response requires the coordinated function of a range of immunochemicals including lymphocytes, cytokines, immunoglobulins, t-cells, b-cells, neutrophils. An immunodeficiency adversely influences the immune response to a viral infection. Every biological component must be present if the immune response/reaction is to proceed satisfactorily! In addition the various immune proteins requires the supply of essential minerals, in particular Magnesium and Zinc, which are essential if they are to function correctly. The accumulation of Mercury in the autistic indicates that the levels of essential minerals, and the regulation of inter-cellular acidity, may have become compromised.

The use of the MMR triple vaccine within the current vaccine schedule appears to inhibit the normal immune response which, directly or indirectly, ultimately leads to chromosomal and/or genetic damage and/or dysfunction. That it occurs mainly in boys indicates that this is a genetic and chromosomal problem. The occurrence of GWS in adults, a condition with many features which are common with autism, indicates the problem may be due to the number and/or intense schedule of vaccinations however this does not excuse the measles or MMR vaccine from suspicion. In scientific research it is normal to look for precedents and/or comparable situations in efforts to establish an explanation. The most obvious link is the larger than normal number of vaccinations which have been administered.

The multiple MMR vaccine appears to raise body temperature creating what is commonly termed a 'fever'. This lowers the prevailing level of immunity and compromises the coherent and coordinated function of the physiological systems. It suggests (1) vaccines given singly may pose less risk than multiple vaccines; (2) the greater the loading of vaccines, the greater will be the amount of genetic changes; (3) some vaccines may pose a greater risk than others e.g. pertussis and measles; (4) the way in which vaccines are administered will be accompanied by different side-effects e.g. if pertussis is followed by measles or vice-versa, if BCG which often gives a beneficial effect is followed by the pertussis vaccine, if vaccines are given in combination, etc; (5) the time between vaccinations; and (6) the time in a child's life when a vaccine is administered will be significant i.e. if before or after the first year. Increased disease loading is the inevitable consequence of multiple vaccine or lots of single vaccines or triple vaccines e.g. of asthma, autoimmune disease, etc. It suggests that adherence to the vaccine schedule is the problem – too many vaccines, too quickly.

Vaccines cause an inflammatory response in some e.g. for those with an inadequately developed or artificially lowered immune system, for those genetically predisposed, or perhaps due to viral or bacterial infection. This creates genetic alterations and/or dysfunction which influences the brain's ability to regulate the physiological systems. It influences the lymphatic system and its ability to excrete Mercury and heavy metals, and lead to long-term damage and problems processing sensory/cognitive input. It influences the autonomic nervous system and the stability of all related physiological systems including temperature, blood pressure, blood cell content, blood glucose, digestion, excretion, sleeping, etc. Further evidence of multi-level dysfunction is evident from unusual brain-wave stability, aberrant sleep patterns, loss of sense perception and coordination, mirror neuron dysfunction, lower pain thresholds, mental and physical deterioration, short periods of concentration, reduction of the visual field, etc. That it is a problem of multi-systemic dysfunction is further supported by noting how sensory therapies can have some effect.

Where is the proof that vaccines are safe? The argument has never been that they are completely safe but that the consequences are less than having the disease. Now it is illustrated that the consequences of intensive vaccination schedules pose a greater risk than could ever have been imagined. Perhaps the cost of managing or treating those with Regressive Autism now exceeds the cost of administering vaccines or the cost of treating the unvaccinateds who contract viral infections.

The overuse of vaccines leads to the evolution of new viral strains (an unsurprising development when the local environment to which it is exposed is being altered by new proteins), structural variants, altered DNA, increased acidity, etc.

Vaccines are an essential component of preventative healthcare however it may be necessary to review the ways in which vaccines are used, administered and regulated (312) i.e. as drugs are tested in the clinical environment to assess their interaction with other drugs. The cumulative use of vaccines including that of multiple vaccines should be researched and shown, through double-blind placebo controlled clinical trials, to be free from any such interactions i.e. of one single vaccine with another single or multiple vaccine or drug. The effect of vaccines should be followed up over a significant period e.g. 2-3 years. It has been considered unethical to select a control group of children which would otherwise would not be vaccinated yet such is the levels of conscientious objectors in the industrialized world and through circumstances of impoverishment in the underdeveloped countries that such statistics must currently exist (20-23, 39-42). There is sufficient evidence which illustrates, at least to those who are sufficiently open-minded to listen, that the unvaccinated have much less exposure to disease.

There is sufficient evidence to illustrate that vaccination should be avoided or delayed in children who have lower levels of immunity. If so, how to assess whether a child has a greater predisposition to an adverse vaccine reaction and the subsequent development of autism? (363) The diagnosis of just one child and hence the prevention of one case of Regressive Autism will lead to a cost-saving of £2.4M (over the life of the child.

The doctor's Hippocratic oath requires that the doctor does not harm the patient. The recent Report (by Robert Francis QC) of the Staffordshire Hospitals NHS Trust Public Enquiry makes clear that harming patient health is no longer to be tolerated and places a legal responsibility on doctors to act in their patient's best interests. If so, perhaps it is time when greater care should be given regarding the administration of vaccinations e.g. giving more time between vaccinations, giving the mumps and rubella vaccinations later in childhood, giving vaccination to children after 6 months, delaying the vaccination schedule in breast-fed mothers, etc. *Who is going to argue that it is better to risk contracting Regressive Autism through vaccination or to risk the effects and side-effects of the disease by natural exposure?* The issue becomes yet more divisive when considering that the process of vaccination does not confer long term immunity (252-255,365). Natural exposure confers lifelong immunity whilst vaccination provides only short term immunity and may predispose to future viral episodes of this and other diseases.

At current rates of occurrence, circa 1 in 100 children, in a population of 60M this will lead to circa 100,000 predominantly male children having to be partially or completely cared-for by the state within a generation at a cost of £240Bn. If we assume a lifespan of just 40 years for such autistics this represents a cost of circa £6Bn pa i.e. an estimated 5-10% of the current cost of running the NHS.

Perhaps we should ask if some vaccines necessary in the industrialized world e.g. (i) if a child in the developed world is no longer exposed to tetanus or polio as a result of changes to lifestyle and better levels of sanitation. With more than 200 other vaccines under development this must be an issue of review. Which vaccines are necessary? (ii) Mumps is sufficiently benign that 40% of people who contract the condition are not aware that they have done so. In addition, as pointed out earlier, the incidence of mumps in South Wales, increased following the measles outbreak and following a much greater uptake of the MMR vaccination. If so, is the mumps vaccination necessary?

The risks from disease and vaccinations differ upon location. In the developed world, there is an estimated 0.0-0.1% risk of mortality from measles which compares with a 0.6% risk and rising (with some estimates at 1-2%) of autism in the developed and developing world markets. This excludes the cost of treating the wide range of side-effects which can be attributed to the use of vaccines. The cost of treating vaccine-related side-effects may now be far greater than the diseases against which the vaccine(s) were designed to protect. Furthermore, in the developed world there is a highly developed social structure which is able to assist parents to deal with the condition. By comparison, what are the implications for an autistic child in the developing world where there is absence of resources to deal with the condition? Having Regressive Autism in the third world may be life-threatening if the parents do not have the resources to care for a vaccine-damaged child. There is a need to protect against disease e.g. in those travelling to and from countries in which the disease is prevalent.

9. Conclusions

The evidence suggests that vaccines are significantly implicated in the occurrence of Regressive Autism. It is suggested that we consider the distinct possibility that vaccines disrupt the genetic profile (mainly that of male infants between 1 and 2 years) and the ability of the brain, perhaps the prefrontal cortex, to regulate the autonomic nervous system and physiological systems. This is manifest as a disruption of a single physiological system or of more than one physiological system. It disrupts the regulation of temperature, pH and other physiological systems and creates an inflammatory response which disrupts the function of the lymphatic system and hence the elimination of mercury and other neurotoxins. Mercury and other metallic neurotoxins accumulate and are manifest as the wide range of physiological and cognitive disorders which are associated with Regressive Autism i.e. the complete disruption of sense perception and coordination, the onset of the range of pathologies outlined in this article, and the almost complete disruption of the quality and quantity of life of those affected.

The complex and emotional nature of the debate is recognised. The parent faces the absolute and unwavering belief by immunologists that vaccines are essential for good health, almost irrespective of the facts including side-effects, yet the financial and social implications of this ever-increasing problem has not yet been fully appreciated. The medical profession must at some stage recognise that they are compromised. Their blind belief in vaccines is being challenged by the recognition that the problem keeps increasing each year They cannot continue to prescribe vaccines if they recognise that vaccines are responsible for the problem. It is a crisis of enormous magnitude and of political and scientific significance. It should not be ignored any longer.

There is a need for a review of vaccine policy, for an impartial cost-benefit analysis of the benefits and costs arising from vaccine use, a projection of future increased occurrence of Regressive Autism and Autistic Spectrum Disorders, and to consider:

- review the dates at which vaccines should be given to children bearing in mind (i) the vulnerability of children, perhaps due to their level of immune development, (ii) of specific populations with suppressed immune function, (iii) whether they are being breast fed and/or the health of the parent i.e. the quality of maternal milk, (iv) the actual longevity of each child e.g. if born prematurely (366);
- review the incidence of Regressive Autism in children below 3 years in Wales in the period 2013-15 to see if the numbers of deaths following vaccination increases; and whether the rate of occurrence of Regressive Autism and Autistic Spectrum Disorders increases during this period;
- review the incidence of Regressive Autism in children below 3 years in England in the period 2013-15 to see if the numbers of deaths following vaccination increases; and if the rate of occurrence of Regressive Autism and Autistic Spectrum Disorders increases during this period;
- establish tests which can determine whether a child has a low level of immunity before the test and/or could be susceptible to the condition;
- review which vaccines are necessary i.e. to remove from the vaccine schedule the vaccines which are not necessary or useful;
- increase the time between vaccinations to enable a child's immune response to recover to a satisfactory level;
- reduce the use of multiple vaccines i.e. to replace multiple vaccines with single vaccines;
- review when vaccines should be administered i.e. during the period when the child's immune response is strongest.

- research whether supplementation with calcipotriol could prevent or reduce the onset of regressive autism;
- eliminate the need for Mercury and Aluminium in vaccines and ensure that the safety limits for heavy metals e.g. mercury and aluminium, are not exceeded by vaccine schedules.
- research how heavy metals, which appear to accumulate in the autistic child, could be eliminated from their systems;
- subject vaccines to the regimen of double-blind clinical studies which follow-up the effect of vaccines over an epidemiologically significant period e.g. into adulthood;

and finally,

- there is a need for genetic studies to track the onset of genetic changes before and after vaccination (some work is believed to have been undertaken at Stanford University although the outcomes are not known and/or have not been published).

In conclusion, it is recognised that the parents of children born in these times face a huge dilemma. It is a dilemma which did not face their parents because regressive autism is a relatively recent phenomena. They have the choice of vaccinating or not vaccinating their 1-2 years child. If they vaccinate and their child develops Regressive Autism they will blame the vaccination but will have little redress for compensation. Moreover, the vaccine manufacturers have been indemnified by governments against claims that vaccines could cause regressive autism. If the parent does not vaccinate they run the risk of side-effects due to contracting disease. If so, they will blame themselves for not vaccinating their child and/or those who have persuaded them not to vaccinate their child.

We are sleep walking into a problem of immense proportions. Something has to be done.

Acknowledgements

We thank the many researchers who through their work have made this article possible. The author hopes that this article will contribute to a wider debate of the issues and will assist parents to make a better decision when dealing with the thorny issue of whether or not to vaccinate their child.

References

(1) Rimland B. The autism increase: research is needed on the vaccine connection. ***Autism Research Review*** 2000;14(1):3,6.

(2) VOSI Research Report RR 12-V50.2A. The Contribution of Mercury, the MMR and DPT Triple Vaccines and Genetics as Causal Factors in Learning Disabilities and Autism. http://www.voicesofsafety.com/ph/v502a/research/

(3) Tuomilehto J, Rewers M, Reunanen A, et al. Increasing trend in type 1 (insulin-dependent)diabetes mellitus in childhood in Finland. Analysis of age, calendar time and birth cohort effects during 1965 to 1984. ***Diabetologia*** 1991;34(4):282-287.

(4) Kelly HA, Russel MT, Jones TW, Byrne GC. Dramatic increase in incidence of insulin dependent diabetes mellitus in Western Australia. ***Med. J. Aust.*** 1994; 161:426-429.

(5) Rewers M, LaPorte RE, Walczak M, Dmochowski K,Bogaczynska E. Apparent epidemic of insulin-dependent diabetes mellitus in Midwestern Poland. ***Diabetes*** 1987;36:106-113.

(6) Barnard J, Broach S, Potter D and Prior A (2002). Autism in Schools: Crisis or Challenge? National Autistic Society. http://www.autism.org.uk/content/1/c4/29/23/aawesn_ew02.pdf

(7) Baird G. Prevalence of disorders of the autism spectrum in a population cohort of children in South Thames: the Special Needs and Autism Project (SNAP). ***The Lancet*** 2006; 368(9531):210-5.

(8) Skuse DH, Mandy W, Steer C, Miller LL, Goodman R, Lawrence K, Emond A, Golding J. Social Communication Competence and Functional Adaptation in a General Population of Children: Preliminary Evidence for Sex-by-Verbal IQ Differential Risk. ***J. Amer. Acad. of Child and Adolescent Psychiatry*** 2009;48(2):128-137.

(9) Altman DG, Bland JM. Absence of evidence is not evidence of absence. ***British Medical Journal*** 1995;311:485.

(10) O'Callaghan FJ. Autism—what is it and where does it come from? ***Q J Med*** 2002; 95: 263-265.

(11) Crabtree GR. Our fragile intellect. Part II. Trends in Genetics 2013;29(1):3-5.

(12) Bainbridge K., Hoffman H, Cowie C. Diabetes and hearing impairment in the United States: Audiometric evidence from the National Health and Nutrition Examination Survey, 1999 to 2004. Annals of Internal Medicine 2008;149, 1–10.

(13) Kruger J, Dunning D. Unskilled and unaware of it: how difficulties in recognizing one's own incompetence lead to inflated self-assessments. ***J. Pers. Soc. Psychol.*** 1999;77(6):1121-34.

(14) Lander E. http://www.pbs.org/wgbh/nova/genome/deco_lander.html

(15) Gottlieb S. US study shows 10-fold increase in autism over the past 20 years ***British Medical Journal*** 2003;326:71

(16) Hertz-Picciotto I, Delwiche L. The Rise in Autism and the Role of Age at Diagnosis. ***Epidemiology*** 2009;20(1):84-90.

(17) Barnevik-Olsson M, Gillberg C, Fernell E. Prevalence of autism in children born to Somali parents living in Sweden: a brief report. ***Dev. Med. Child Neurol.*** 2008;50(8):598-601.

(18) http://www.cdc.gov/media/releases/2012/p0329_autism_disorder.html

(19) Gillberg C, Coleman M. *The Biology of the Autistic Syndromes - 2nd Edition, page 90.* Mac Keith Press, 1992

(20) Olmsted D. http://www.nomercury.org/science/documents/Articles/UPI-The_Age_of_Autism-Mercury_and_the_Amish_5-21-05.pdf;

(21) Olmsted D. http://www.whale.to/vaccine/olmsted.html;

(22) Olmsted D. http://www.upi.com/Consumer_Health_Daily/Reports/2006/07/28/the_age_of_autism_amish_bill_introduced/3532/;

(23) Olmsted D. http://pittsburgh.indymedia.org/news/2005/06/18948.php

(24) Bailey A, Phillips W, Rutter M. Autism: Towards an Integration of Clinical, Genetic, Neuro-psychological, and Neurobiological Perspectives. ***J. Child Psychol. Psychiatry*** 1996;37(1):89-126.

(25) Filipek P, Accardo P, Baranek G, Cook E, Dawson G, Gordon B, Gravel J, Johnson C, Kallen R, Levy S, Minshew N, Prizant B, Rapin I, Rogers S, Stone W, Teplin S, Tuchman R, Volkmar F. The Screening and Diagnosis of Autistic Spectrum Disorders. ***J. Autism and Dev. Disord.*** 1999;29(6):439-484.

(26) Baranek G. Autism During Infancy: A Retrospective Video Analysis of Sensory-Motor and Social Behaviors and 9-12 Months of Age. ***J. Autism and Dev. Disord.*** 1999;29(3):213-224.

(27) Lewine JD, Andrews R, Chez M, Patil A-A, Devinsky O, Smith M, Kanner A, Davis JT, Funke M, Jones G, Chong B, Provencal S, Weisend M, Lee RR, Orrison WW. Magnetoenchalography in Children with an Autistic Epileptiform Regression. ***J. Pediatrics*** 1999;405-418.

(28) Goldberg WA, Osann K, Filipek PA, Laulhere T, Jarvis K, Modahl C, Flodman P, Spence MA. Language and other Regression: Assessment and Timing. Journal of Autism and Developmental Disorders 2003;33(6):607-616.

(29) Montinari M, Favoino B, Roberto A. Role of Immunogenetics in the Diagnosis of Postvaccinal CNS Pathology. Presented in Naples, May 9, 1996. Associazione per la Libera Universita Internazionale de Medicina Omeopatica "Samuel Hahnemann" (LUIMO). http://www.healthy.net/library/articles/coulter/biochem.htm

(30) Furlano RI, Anthony A, Day R, Brown A, McGarvey L, Thomson MA, Davies SE, Berelowitz M, Forbes A, Wakefield AJ, Walker-Smith JA, Murch SH. Colonic CD8 and gamma delta T-cell infiltration with epithelial damage in children with autism. ***J. Pediatr.*** 2001;138(3):366-72.
(31) Kurita H. Infantile autism with speech loss before the age of thirty months. ***Journal of the American Academy of Child Psychiatry*** 1985;24(2):191-196.
(32) Jarbrink K, Knapp M. The Economic Impact of Autism in Britain. ***Autism*** 2001;5(1):7-22.
(33) Crabtree G. MedicineNet November 16, 2012
(34) http://www.independent.co.uk/life-style/health-and-families/health-news/italian-court-reignites-mmr-vaccine-debate-after-award-over-child-with-autism-7858596.html?origin=internalSearch
(35) Medical Research Council (2002) Review of Autism Research: Causes and Epidemiology, MRC: London
(36) http://www.ageofautism.com/2011/05/vaccines-and-autism-what-do-epidemiological-studies-really-tell-us.html
(37) Wong CCY, Meaburn EL, Ronald A, Price TS, Jeffries AR, Schalkwyk LC, Plomin R, Mill J. Methylomic analysis of monozygotic twins discordant for autism spectrum disorder and related behavioural traits. Molecular Psychiatry advance online publication, April 23 2013. doi:10.1038/mp.2013.41
(38) Palmer RF, Blanchard S, Stein Z, Mandell D, Miller C. Environmental mercury release, special education rates, and autism disorder: an ecological study of Texas. ***Health & Place.*** 2006;12(2):203–209.
(39) Bachmair A. www.vaccineinjury.info. Vaccine Free. 111 Stories of Unvaccinated Children. ISBN 978-147839529.
(40) Nederlands Vereniging Kritisch Prikken 2004 Survey Findings (reproduced in reference 45)
(41) http://educate-yourself.org/vcd/califoregonunvaccinatedchildrensurvey03nov07.shtml
November 3, 2007
(42) http://www.generationrescue.org/survey.html California-Oregon Unvaccinated Children Survey Links Vaccines & Autism (Nov. 3, 2007)
(43) Cherry JD, Mortimer EA. Acellular and whole-cell pertussis vaccines in Japan: a report of a visit by US scientists. ***JAMA*** 1987;257:1375.
(44) Letai AG, Snyder KM, Fett JD, et al. Smallpox and smallpox vaccination. ***N. Engl J. Med.*** 2002;347:691-2.
(45) McDonald KL, Huq SI, Lix LM, Becker AB, Kozyrskyi AL. Delay in diphtheria, pertussis, tetanus vaccination is associated with a reduced risk of childhood asthma. ***Journal of Allergy and Clinical Immunology*** 2008;121(3):626-631
(46) Enriquez R, Addington W, Davis F, Freels S, Park CL, Hershow RC, Persky V, The relationship between vaccine refusal and self-report of atopic disease in children. ***Journal of Allergy and Clinical Immunology*** 2005;115(4):737-744.
(47) Glanz JM, Newcomer SR, Narwaney KJ, Hambidge SJ, Daley MF, Wagner NM, McClure DL, Xu S, Rowhani-Rahbar A, Lee GM, Nelson JC, Donahue JG, Naleway AL, Nordin JD, Lugg MM, Weintraub ES. A Population-Based Cohort Study of Undervaccination in 8 Managed Care Organizations Across the United States ***JAMA Pediatr.*** 2013;():1-8. doi:10.1001/jamapediatrics.2013.502.
(48) Miller NZ, Goldman GS. Infant mortality rates regressed against number of vaccine doses routinely given: Is there a biochemical or synergistic toxicity? ***Hum. Exp. Toxicol.*** 2011 September;30(9):1420–1428.
(49) Classen DC, Classen JB. The timing of pediatric immunization and the risk of insulin- dependent diabetes. ***Infectious Diseases in Clinical Practice*** 1997;6:449-454.
(50) Classen JB. Discontinuation of BCG Vaccination Precedes Significant Drop in Type 2 Diabetes in Japanese Children. Role of Inflammation and Cortisol Activity as a Cause of Type 2 Diabetes. ***The Open Endocrinology Journal*** 2008;2:1-4.
(51) Classen JB, Classen DC. Association between type 1 diabetes and Hib vaccine, causal relation likely. ***British Medical Journal*** 1999;319:1133.
(52) Classen JB, Classen DC. Clustering of cases of insulin dependent diabetes (IDDM) occurring three years after Hemophilus influenza B (HiB) immunization support causal relationship between immunization and IDDM. ***Autoimmunity*** 2002;35:247-253
(53) Classen JB. Diabetes epidemic follows hepatitis B immunization program. ***New Zealand Medical Journal*** 1996;109:195.
(54) Pozzilli P, Visalli N, Coppolino G, Classen DC, Classen JB and the IMDIAB Group. Hepatitis B Vaccine Associated with an Increased Risk of Type 1 Diabetes in Italy. Abstract 272, 60th Scientific Session, ***American Diabetes Association*** Meeting, San Antonio, Texas: June 13, 2000.
(55) Classen JB, Classen DC. Clustering of Cases of Type 1 Diabetes Mellitus Occurring 2-4 Years After Vaccination is Consistent with Clustering After Infections and Progression to Type I Diabetes Mellitus in Autoantibody Positive Individuals. ***J.Pediatric Endocrinology & Metabolism*** 2003;16:495-508.
(56) McCarthy N, Weintraub E, Vellozzi C, Duffy J, Gee J, Donahue JG, Jackson ML, Lee GM, Glanz J, Baxter R, Lugg MM, Naleway A, Omer SB, Nakasato C, Vazquez-Benitez G, DeStefano F. Mortality Rates and Cause-of-Death Patterns in a Vaccinated Population. ***American Journal of Preventive Medicine*** 2013;45(1): doi: 10.1016/j.amepre.2013.02.020.

(57) Obomsawin R. http://www.whale.to/vaccine/ImmunizationGraphs-RO2009.pdf
(58) Honda H, Shimizu Y, Rutter M. No effect of MMR withdrawal on the incidence of autism: a total population study. ***Journal of Child Psychology and Psychiatry*** 2005;46(6):572-9.
(59) http://www.newscientist.com/data/images/ns/cms/dn7076/dn7076-1_572.jpg
(60) Gallagher CM, Goodman MS. Hepatitis B vaccination of male neonates and autism diagnosis, NHIS 1997-2002. ***J. Toxicol. Environ. Health A.*** 2010;73(24):1665-77.
(61) Takahashi H, Suzumura S, et al. An epidemiological study on Japanese Autism concerning Routine Childhood Immunization History. ***Jpn. J. Infectious Disease*** 2003;56:114-7.
(62) Julia P. Owen, Elysa J. Marco, Shivani Desai, Emily Fourie, Julia Harris, Susanna S. Hill, Anne B. Arnett, Pratik Mukherjee. **Abnormal white matter microstructure in children with sensory processing disorders**. *NeuroImage: Clinical*, 2013; DOI: 10.1016/j.nicl.2013.06.009
(63) Ewing GW, Ewing EN. Cognition, the Autonomic Nervous System and the Physiological Systems. ***Biogenic Amines*** 2008;22(3):140-163.
(64) Ewing GW, Parvez SH. The influence of Pathologies and EEG frequencies upon sense perception and coordination in Developmental Dyslexia. A Unified Theory of Developmental Dyslexia. ***N.Am.J.Med.Sci.*** 2012;4(3):109-116.
(65) Duffy FH, Als H. A stable pattern of EEG spectral coherence distinguishes children with autism from neuro-typical controls - a large case control study. ***BMC Medicine*** (26 June 2012), 10:64 doi:10.1186/1741-7015-10-64.
(66) Mutter J, Naumann J, Schneider R, Walach H, Haley B. Mercury and autism: accelerating evidence? ***NeuroEndocrinol Lett.*** 2005 Oct;26(5):439-46.
(67) Geier DA, King PG, Sykes LK, Geier MR. A comprehensive review of mercury provoked autism. ***Indian J. Med. Res.*** 2008;128(4):383-411.
(68) Bernard S, Enayati A, Redwood L, Roger H, Binstock T. Autism: a novel form of mercury poisoning. ***Med. Hypotheses*** 2001;56(4)462-471.
(69) Bolton PF, Carcani-Rathwell I, Hutton J, Goode S, Howlin P, Rutter M. Epilepsy in autism: features and correlates. ***The British Journal of Psychiatry*** 2011;198:289-294.
(70) Horvath K, Papadimitriou JC, Rabsztyn A, Drachenberg C, Tyson Tildon J. Gastrointestinal abnormalities in children with autistic disorder. The ***Journal of Pediatrics*** November 1999; 135(5):559-63.
(71) Torrente F, Anthony A, Heuschkel RB, Thomson MA, Ashwood P, Murch SH. Focal-Enhanced Gastritis in Regressive Autism with Features Distinct from Crohn's and Helicobacter Pylori Gastritis. ***American Journal of Gastroenterology*** 2004;598-605.
(72) Malow B, Adkins KW, McGrew SW, Wang L, Goldman SE, Fawkes D, Burnette C. Melatonin for sleep in children with autism: a controlled trial examining dose, tolerability, and outcomes. ***J. Autism and Dev. Disord.*** 2012;42(8):1729-37.
(73) Johnson CR, Turner KS, et al. Comparison of sleep questionnaires in the assessment of sleep disturbances in children with autism spectrum disorders. ***Sleep Medicine*** 2012;13(7):795-801.
(74) http://www.snoezeleninfo.com/whatIsSnoezelen.asp
(75) Mayo J, Chlebowski C, Eigsti IM, Fein, D. Age of first words predicts cognitive ability and adaptive skills in children with ASD. ***J. Autism and Dev. Disord.*** 2012 Advance online publication. doi: 10.1007/s10803-012-1558-02012.
(76) Heuer L, Ashwood P, Schauer J, Goines P, Krakowiak P, Hertz-Picciotto I, Hansen R, Croen LA, Pessah IN, van de Water J. Reduced Levels of Immunoglobulin in Children With Autism Correlates With Behavioral Symptoms. ***Autism Res.*** 2008 October 1; 1(5): 275–283.
(77) http://www.fountia.com/autism/medical-treatment
(78) Infectious Diseases Society of America December 16, 2011
(79) Vashisht N, Puliyel J. Introducing pentavalent vaccine in the EPI in India: A counsel for caution ***Indian Journal of Medical Ethics*** 2010;132:1-3.
(80) ***MMWR*** 1997; 32[29]: 384-385.
(81) Partinen M, Saarenpaa-Heikkila O, Ilveskoski I, Hublin C, Linna M, Olsen P, Nokelainen RA, Espo M, Rusanen H, Olme J, Satila H, Arikka H, Kaipanen P, Julkunen I, Kirjvainen T. Increased Incidence and Clinical Picture of Childhood Narcolepsy after 2009 H1N1 Pandemic Vaccination Campaign in Finland. ***PLoS One*** 2012;7(3):e33723.
(82) Vaccine May 31, 2012 [Epub ahead of print]
(83) Solomon T, Kneen R, Dung NM. Polio-like illness due to Japanese encephalitis virus ***The Lancet*** 1998;351:1094-97.
(84) Fındık A,Çiftci A. Bacterial DNA Vaccines in Veterinary Medicine: a Review. ***Journal of Veterinary Advances*** 2012;2(4):139-148.
(85) Evans DMA, Dunn G, Minor PD, Schild GC, Cann AJ, Stanway G, Almond JW, Currey K, Maizel JV. Increased neurovirulence associated with a single nucleotide change in a noncoding region of the Sabin type 3 poliovirus genome. ***Nature*** 1985;314:548-550.
(86) Noakes TD, St Clair Gibson A, Lambert EV. From Catastrophe to Complexity: A novel model of Integrative Central Neural Regulation of Effort and Fatigue During Exercise in Humans: Summary and Conclusions. ***British***

Journal of Sports Medicine 2005;39(2):120–124.(87) Noakes TD, Peltonen JE, Rusko HK. Evidence that a central governor regulates exercise performance during acute hypoxia and hyperoxia. ***The Journal of Experimental Biology*** 2001;204 (Pt 18): 3225–3234.

(88) Toraldo R, Tolone C, Catalanotti C, Ianiello R, D'Avanzo M, Canino G, Galdiero F, Iafusco F. Effect of Measles-Mumps-Rubella Vaccination on Polymorphonuclear Neutrophil Function in Children. ***ACTA Pediatrics*** 1992;81:887-90.

(89) Mostafa GA, Al-Ayadhi LY. Reduced serum concentrations of 25-hydroxy vitamin D in children with autism: Relation to autoimmunity. ***Journal of Neuroinflammation*** 2012;9:201.

(90) Grant WB, Cannell JJ. Autism prevalence in the United States with respect to solar UV-B doses: An ecological study. ***Dermato-Endocrinology*** 2013;5(1):1-6.

(91) Jackson KM, Nazar AM. Breastfeeding, the Immune Response, and Long-term Health. ***J. Am. Osteopath. Assoc.*** 2006;106(4):203-207

(92) Barbur JL. ***Trends in Cognitive Sciences*** 2003;7(10):434-436 Understanding colour: Normal and Defective Colour Vision edited by J.D. Mollon, J. Pokorny and K. Knoblauch, ISBN 0-19-852530-3.

(93) Muntoni S, Serra A, Mascia C, Songini M. Dyschromatopsia in diabetes mellitus and its relation to metabolic control. ***Diabetes Care*** 1982;5(4):375-378.

(94) Lloyd MJ, Fraunfelder FW. Drug-induced optic neuropathies. ***Drugs Today*** 2007; 43(11):827.

(95) Martinek K, Berezin I. Artificial Light-Sensitive Enzymatic Systems as Chemical Amplifiers of Weak Light Signals. ***Photochemistry and Photobiology*** 1979;29:637-649.

(96) Azeemi STY, Raza SM, Yasinzai M. Colors as Catalysts in Enzymatic Reactions. ***J.Acupuncture and Meridian Studies*** 2008;1(2):139-142.

(97) Kipnis J, Cohen H, Cardon M, Ziv Y, Schwartz M. T cell deficiency leads to cognitive dysfunction: Implications for therapeutic vaccination for schizophrenia and other psychiatric conditions. ***Proc. Natl. Acad. Sci. USA.*** 2004;101(21):8180–8185.

(98) Grakov, I. *Strannik Diagnostic and Treatment System; a Virtual Scanner for the Health Service.* Minutes of Meeting No. 11 of the Presidium of the Siberian of the Academy of Medical Sciences of the USSR (AMN) 14, held in Novosibirsk 4 December 1985.

(99) Grakov, I. *Description of Virtual Scanning System for Operators.* Mimex, Sochi, Russia: 2002. English translation available at: http://www.montague-diagnostics.co.uk/files/Grakov/Article7.pdf

(100) Cox RH, Shealy CN, Cady RK, Liss S. ***The Journal of Neurological and Orthopaedic Medicine and Surgery*** 1996;17:32-34.

(101) Bower B. Perception may dance to the beat of collective neuronal rhythms. ***Science News*** 1998;153(8):120.

(102) Milne E, Scope A, Pascalis O, Buckley D, Makeig S. Independent Component Analysis Reveals Atypical Electroencephalographic Activity during Visual Perception in Individuals with Autism. ***Biological Psychiatry*** 2009;65(1):22-30.

(103) Varela F.J. http://findarticles.com/p/articles/mi_m1200/is_8_155/ai_54062666

(104) Baron-Cohen S. Is There a Normal Phase of Synaesthesia in Development? ***Psyche*** 1996;2(27).

(105) Baron-Cohen S, Wyke M, Binnie C. Hearing words and seeing colours: an experimental investigation of a case of synaesthesia. ***Perception*** 1987;16:761-67.

(106) Baron-Cohen S, Harrison J, Goldstein L, Wyke M. Coloured speech perception: Is synaesthesia what happens when modularity breaks down? ***Perception*** 1993;22:419-426.

(107) Miltner WHR, Braun C, Arnold M, Witte H, Taub E. Coherence of gamma- band EEG activity as a basis for Associative Learning. ***Nature*** 1999;397:434-436.

(108) Hardan AY, Keshavan MS, Sucheeta S, Velumapalli M, Minshew NJ. An MRI study of minor physical anomalies in autism. ***J. Autism Dev. Disord.*** 2006;36:607-611.

(109) Minshew NJ, Williams DL. The New Neurobiology of Autism: Cortex, Connectivity, and Neuronal Organization. ***Arch. Neurol.***. 2007;64(7):945-950.

(110) Kennedy DP, Courchesne E. The intrinsic functional organization of the brain is altered in autism. ***Neuroimage*** 2008;39(4):1877-85.

(111) Curran LK, Newschaffer CJ, Lee L-C, Crawford SO, Johnston MV, Zimmerman AW. Behaviors Associated With Fever in Children With Autism Spectrum Disorders. ***Pediatrics*** 2007;120(6):e1386-e1392.

(112) Courchesne E. New evidence of cerebellar and brainstem hypoplasia in autistic infants, children, and adolescents: The MRI imaging study by Hashimoto and colleagues. ***J. Autism and Dev. Disord.*** 1995;25:19-22.

(113) Bower JM, Parsons L. Rethinking the Lesser Brain. ***Scientific American*** 2003;289:50-57.

(114) Ritvo ER, Freeman BJ, Scheibel AB, Duong T, Robinson H, Guthrie D, Ritvo A. Lower Purkinje cell counts in the cerebella of four autistic subjects: intitial findings of the UCLA-NSAC Autopsy Research Report, ***American Journal of Psychiatry*** 1986;143:862-866.

(115) Hashimoto T, Tayama M, Miyazaki M, Sakurama N, Yoshimoto T, Murakawa K, Kuroda Y. Reduced brainstem size in children with autism. ***Brain & Development*** 1992;14(2):94-97.

(116) Hashimoto T, Tayama M, Murakawa K, Yoshimoto T, Miyazaki M, Harada M, Kuroda Y. Development of the brainstem and cerebellum in autistic patients. ***J. Autism and Dev. Disord.*** 1995;25(1):1-18.
(117) Ewing.GW. and Ewing EN. 'Virtual Scanning – a new generation of medical technology – beyond biomedicine?' ISBN 978-0-9556213-0-7 pub Montague Healthcare books.
(118) Krakov SV. Colour Vision and the Autonomic Nervous System. ***Journal of the Optical Society of America J. Opt. Soc. Am***. 1941;31:335-337.
(119) Cumberland P, Rahi J.S, Peckham CS. Impact of congenital colour vision on education and unintentional injuries: findings from the 1958 British Birth Cohort. ***British Medical Journal*** 2004;329:1074-5.
(120) Van De Geijn EJ, Tukkie R, Van Philips LAM, Punt H. Bilateral optic neuritis with branch retinal artery occlusion associated with vaccination. ***Documenta Ophthalmologica*** 1994;86(4):403-408.
(121) Sigman M, Ungerer JA, Mundy P, Sherman T. Cognition in Autistic Children. ***Handbook of Autism and Pervasive Developmental Disorders***, John Wiley & Sons, Inc., 1987, pp 103-130.
(122) O'Neill M, Jones RSP. Sensory-Perceptual Abnormalities in Autism: A Case For More Research? ***J. Autism and Dev. Disord.*** 1997;27(3):283-293.
(123) Takayanagi Y, Yoshida M, Bielsky IF, Ross HE, Kawamata M, Onaka T, Yanagisawa T, Kimura T, Matzuk MM, Young LJ, Nishimori K. Pervasive social deficits, but normal parturition, in oxytocin receptor-deficient mice. ***Proc. Natl. Acad. Sci. USA*** 2005;102:16096-101.
(124) Bartz JA, Hollander E. Oxytocin and experimental therapeutics in autism spectrum disorders. ***Prog. Brain. Res.*** 2008;170:451–62.
(125) Zak PJ, Stanton AA, Ahmadi A. Oxytocin increases generosity in humans. ***PLoS One*** 2007;2(11):e1128.
(126) Panksepp J. Commentary on the possible role of oxytocin in autism. ***J. Autism and Dev. Disord.*** 1993;23(3):567-569.
(127) Porges SW. The Polyvagal Theory: phylogenetic contributions to social behaviour. ***J. Physiol. Behav.*** 2003;79:503-513.
(128) Ewing GW, Parvez SH. Systemic Regulation of Metabolic Function. ***Biogenic Amines*** 2008; 22(6):179-194.
(129) Ewing GW, Ewing EN. NeuroRegulation of the Physiological Systems by the Autonomic Nervous System – their relationship to Insulin Resistance and Metabolic Syndrome. ***Biogenic Amines*** 2008;22;4-5:99-130.
(130) Ewing GW, Parvez SH. The Regulatory Significance of the Autonomic Nervous System and the Physiological Systems, and their relationship to Dyslexia. ***Biogenic Amines*** 2009;23(3):115-190.
(131) Ming X, Julu POO, Brimacombe M, Connor S, Daniels ML. Reduced cardiac parasympathetic activity in children with autism. ***Brain and Development*** 2005;27(7):509-516.
(132) Ashwood P, Van de Water JA. A review of autism and the immune response. ***Clin. Develop. Immunology*** 2004; 11(2);165-174.
(133) Zahn TP, Rumsey JM, Van Kammen DP. Autonomic nervous system activity in autistic, schizophrenic, and normal men: Effects of stimulus significance. ***Journal of Abnormal Psychology*** 1987;96(2):135-144.
(134) Hutt C, Forrest SJ, Richer J. Cardiac Arrhythmia and Behaviour in Autistic Children. ***Acta Psychiatrica Scandinavica*** 2007;51(5):361-372.
(135) Stores G, Wiggs L. Abnormal sleeping patterns associated with autism: a brief review of research findings, assessment methods and treatment strategies. ***Autism*** 1998;2(2):157-170.
(136) Williams PG, Sears LL, Allard A-M. Sleep problems in children with autism. ***Journal of Sleep research*** 2004;13(3):265-268.
(137) Malow BA. Sleep disorders, epilepsy, and autism. ***Mental Retardation and Developmental Disabilities Research Reviews*** 2004;10(2):122-125.
(138) Chugani DC, Sundram BS, Behen M, Lee ML, Moore GJ. Evidence of altered energy metabolism in autistic children. ***Prog. Neuropsychopharmacol. Biol. Psychiatry*** 1999; 23(4):635-41.
(139) Ohnishi T, Matsuda H, Hashimoto T, Kunihiro *T*; Nishikawa M; Uema *T*; Sasaki M. Abnormal blood flow in brain regions. ***Brain*** 2000;123:1838-44.
(140) Starkstein SE, Vazquez S, Vrancic D, Nanclares V, Manes F, Piven J, Plebst C. SPECT findings in mentally retarded autistic individuals. ***J. Neuropsychiatry Clin. Neurosci.*** 2000;12(3):370-5.
(141) Ryu YH, Lee JD, Yoon PH, Kim DI, Lee HB, Shin YJ. Perfusion impairments in infantile autism on technetium-99m ethyl cysteinate dimer brain single-photon emission tomography: comparison with findings on magnetic resonance imaging. ***Eur. J. Nucl. Med.*** 1999;26:253-9.
(142) Jones W, Carr K, Klin A. Absence of preferential looking to the eyes of approaching adults predicts level of social disability in 2-year-olds with autism. ***Archives of General Psychiatry*** 2008;65(8):946-54.
(143) Cascio C, McGlone F, Folger S, Tannan V, Baranek G, Pelphrey KA, Essick G. Tactile Perception in Adults with Autism: a Multidimensional Psychophysical Study. ***J. Autism Dev. Disord.*** 2008;38(1): 127-137.
(144) Rosenhall U, Johansson E, Gillberg C. Oculomotor findings in autistic children. ***Journal of Laryngology and Otology*** 1988;102:435-439.
(145) Rosenhall U, Nordin V, Sandstrom M, Ahlsen G, Gillberg C. Autism and Hearing Loss. ***J. Autism and Dev. Disord.*** 1999;29(5):349-358.

(146) Paulesu E, Harrison J, Baron-Cohen S, Watson JDG, Goldstein L, Heather J, Frackowiak RSJ, Frith CD. The physiology of coloured hearing A PET activation study of colour-word synaesthesia. ***Brain*** 1995;118:661-676.
(147) Grice SJ, Spratling MW, Karmiloff-Smith A, Halit H, Csibra G, de Haan M, Johnson MH. Disordered visual processing and oscillatory brain activity in autism and Williams Syndrome. ***Neuroreport*** 2001;12(12):2697-2700.
(148) Motomi T, Yoko K. Autistic adolescents' autonomic response to mental load. ***Japanese Journal of Child and Adolescent Psychiatry*** 1999;40(4):319-328.
(149) http://www.who.int/bulletin/volumes/86/2/07-040089/en/
(150) McKeown T. The Role of Medicine: Dream, Mirage or Nemesis? Pub: Blackwell, Oxford 1979.
(151) UK Office for National Statistics, 1997; Mortality Statistics: Deaths registered in England & Wales.
(152) Vital Statistics of the United States 1937-1960; Historican Statistics of the United States: Colonial Times to 1970 part 1 Chapter B. Vital Statistics Health & Medical Care pp44-86.
(153) Cohen AD, Shoenfeld Y. Vaccine-induced Autoimmunity. ***Journal of Autoimmunity*** 1996; 9(6): 699-703.
(154) Howson CP, Katz M, Johnston RB, Fineberg HV. Chronic arthritis after rubella vaccination. ***Clin. Infect. Dis.*** 1992;15(2):307-312.
(155) Howson CP, Fineberg HV. Adverse events following pertussis and rubella vaccines. ***JAMA*** 1992;267(3):393-397.
(156) Rook GAW, Stanford JL. Give us this day our daily germs. ***Immunology Today*** 1998; 19:113-116.
(157) Taylor-Robinson AW. Multiple vaccination effects on atopy. ***Allergy*** 1999;54:398-399.
(158) Odent M.R, Culpin E.E, Kimmel T. Pertussis vaccination and asthma: is there a link? ***JAMA*** 1994:272:592-3.
(159) Kemp T, Pearce N, Fitzharris P, Crane J, Fergusson D, St George I, Wickens K, Beasley R. Is Infant Immunisation a risk factor for childhood asthma or allergy? ***Epidemiology*** 1997;8(6):678-80.
(160) Hurwitz EL, Morgenstern H. Effects of diphtheria-tetanus-pertussis or tetanus vaccination on allergies and allergy-related respiratory symptoms among children and adolescents in the United States, ***Journal of Manipulative and Physiological Therapeutics*** 2000;23(2):81-90.
(161) Patel NC, Hertel P, Estes M, Dela Morena M, Noroski L, Revell P, Hanson I, Paul M, Rosenblatt H, Abramson S. Vaccine-acquired rotavirus infection in two infants with severe combined immunodeficiency. ***American Academy of Allergy, Asthma & Immunology*** 2009; Abstract L29.
(162) Cherry JD, Brunell PA, Golden GS, Karzon DT. Report on the Task Force on Pertussis and Pertussis Immunization. ***Pediatrics*** 1988 (81) Supplement.
(163) Terpstra GK, Raaijmakers JA, Kreukniet J. Comparison of vaccination of mice and rats with Haemophilus influenzae and Bordetta pertussis as models of atopy. ***Clin. Exp. Pharmacol. Physiol.*** 1979;6(2):139-49.
(164) Schreurs AJ, Nijkamp FP. Bronchial hyperreactivity to histamine induced by Haemophilus influenzae vaccination. ***Agents Actions*** 1984;15(3-4):211-5.
(165) ***MMWR*** September 06, 1996 / 45(RR-12);1-35. Update: Vaccine Side Effects, Adverse Reactions, Contraindications, and Precautions Recommendations of the Advisory Committee on Immunization Practices (ACIP).
(166) Vertes C, Gonczy S, Lendvay N, Debreczeni LA. A model for experimental asthma provocation in guinea-pigs immunized with Bordetella pertussis. ***Bull Eur. Physiopathol. Respir.*** 1987;23 Suppl 10:111s-113s.
(167) Schreurs AJ, Terpstra GK, Raaijmakers JA, Nijkamp FP. The effects of Haemophilus influenzae vaccination on anaphylactic mediator release and isoprenaline-induced inhibition of mediator release. ***Eur. J. Pharmacol*** 1980;62(4):261-8 .
(168) Bradford Hill A, Knoweldon J. Inoculation and Poliomyelitis. ***British Medical Journal*** 1950; 1-6.
(169) Imani F, Kehoe KE. Infection of Human B Lymphocytes with MMR Vaccine Induces IgE Class Switching. ***J. Clinical Immunology*** 2001;100(3):355-361.
(170) Shields RL, Lai J, Keck R, O'Connell L.Y, Hong K, Meng YG, Weikert SHA, Presta LG. Lack of Fucose on Human IgG1 N-Linked Oligosaccharide Improves Binding to Human Fc RIII and Antibody-dependent Cellular Toxicity. ***J. Biol. Chem.*** 2002; 277(30): 26733-26740.
(171) Kaplan KM, Marder DC, Cochi SL, Preblud SR. Further evidence of the changing epidemiology of a childhood vaccine-preventable disease. ***Journal of the American Medical Association*** 1988;260(10):1434-1438.
(172) Singh VK, Lin SX, Newell E, Nelson C. Abnormal measles-mumps-rubella antibodies and CNS autoimmunity in children with autism. ***Journal of Biomedical Science*** *2002; 9:359-364.*
(173) Mooi FR, van Oirschot H, Heuvelman K, van der Heide HG, Gaastra W, Willems RJ. Olymorphism in the Bordella Pertussis virulence factors P.69/pertactin and pertussis toxin in the Netherlands: temporal trends and evidence for vaccine-driven evolution. ***Infect. Immun.*** 1998;66:670-5.
(174) Gzyl A, Augustynowicz E, van Loo I, Slusarczyk J. Temporal nucleotide changes in pertactin and pertussis toxin genes in *Bordetella pertussis* strains isolated from clinical cases in Poland. ***Vaccine*** 2001;20:299-303.
(175) Ribeiro GS, Reis JN, Cordeiro SM, Lima JB, Gouveia EL, Petersen M, Salgado K, Silva HR, Zanella RC, Almeida SC, Brandileone MC, Reis MG, Ko AI. Prevention of Haemophilus influenzae type b (Hib) meningitis and emergence of serotype replacement with type a strains after introduction of Hib immunization in Brazil. ***J. Infect. Dis.*** 2003;187(1):109-16.

(176) Litt DJ, Neal SE, Fry NK. Changes in Genetic Diversity of the *Bordetella pertussis* Population in the United Kingdom between 1920 and 2006 Reflect Vaccination Coverage and Emergence of a Single Dominant Clonal Type. ***Journal of Clinical Microbiology*** 2009;47(3):680-688.
(177) Tsang RS, Sill ML, Skinner SJ, Law DK, Zhou J, Wylie J. Characterization of invasive Haemophilus influenzae disease in Manitoba, Canada, 2000-2006: invasive disease due to non-type b strains. ***Clin. Infect. Dis.*** 2007;44(12):1611-4.
(178) Nahm MH, Lin J, Finkelstein JA, Pelton SI. Increase in the Prevalence of the Newly Discovered Pneumococcal Serotype 6C in the Nasopharynx after Introduction of Pneumococcal Conjugate Vaccine. ***J. Infect. Dis.*** 2009;199:320–325.
(179) Guris D, Strebel PM, Bardenheier B, Brennan M, Tachdjian R, Finch E, Wharton M, Livengood JR. Changing epidemiology of pertussis in the United States: increasing reported incidence among adolescents and adults, 1990-1996. ***Clin. Infect. Dis.*** 1999;28:1230-1237.
(180) Cherry JD. Epidemiological, clinical, and laboratory aspects of pertussis in adults. ***Clin. Infect. Dis.*** 1999; 28(Suppl 2):S112-7.
(181) Huisman W. Vaccine-induced enhancement of viral infections. ***Vaccine*** 2009;27(4): 505-512.
(182) Exley RM, Shaw J, Mowe E, Sun Y-H, West NP, Williamson M, Botto M, Smith H & Tang CM. Available carbon source influences the resistance of *Neisseria meningitidis* against complement. ***J. Exp. Med.*** 2005;16;201(10):1637–1645.
(183) Classen, J.B., and Classen, D.C. Public should be told that vaccines may have adverse effects. ***British Medical Journal*** 1999;318:193.
(184) Stewart GT. Vaccination against whooping-cough. Efficacy versus risks. ***The Lancet*** 1977;1(8005):234-7.
(185) Colville A, Pugh S, Miller E, Schmitt HJ, Just M, Neiss A. Withdrawal of a mumps vaccine. ***Eur. J. Pediatr.*** 1994;153(6):467–8.
(186) Schlegel M, Osterwalder JJ, Galeazzi RL, Vernazza PL. Comparative efficacy of three mumps vaccines during disease outbreak in eastern Switzerland: cohort study. ***British Medical Journal*** 1999;319(7206):352.
(187) Peltola H, Kulkarni PS, Kapre SV, Paunio M, Jadhav SS, Dhere RM. Mumps outbreaks in Canada and the United States: Time for new thinking on mumps vaccines. ***Clin. Infect. Dis.*** 2007;45:459–66.
(188) EPI Newsl. 1980 Feb;2(1):6. Live attenuated measles vaccine.
(189) Rima B.K, Earle J.A, Yeo R.P, Herlihy L, Baczko K, ter Meulen V, Carabaña J, Caballero M, Celma ML, Fernandez-Muñoz R. Temporal and geographical distribution of measles virus genotypes. ***J. Gen. Virol.*** 1995;76(5):1173–80.
(190) Garenne M, Leroy O, Beau J.P, Sene I. Child mortality after high-titre measles vaccines: prospective study in Senegal. ***The Lancet*** 1991;338(8772):903-7.
(191) Trollfors B, Taranger J, Lagergard T, Lind L, Sundh V, Zackrisson G, Lowe CU, Blackwelder W, Robbins JB. A placebo-controlled trial of a pertussis-toxoid vaccine. ***N. Engl. J. Med.*** 1995;333:1045-50.
(192) Marwick C. Acellular pertussis vaccine hailed for infants. ***JAMA*** 1995;274:446-7.
(193) Miller E. Overview of recent clinical trials of acellular pertussis vaccines. ***Biologicals*** 1999;27:79-86.
(194) Torch WC. Diphtheria-pertussis-tetanus (DPT) immunization: a potential cause of the sudden infant death syndrome (SIDS). American Academy of Neurology, 34th Annual Meeting, Apr 25-May 1, 1982. ***Neurology*** 1982;32(4): pt. 2.
(195) Shoenfeld Y, Aron-Maor A. Vaccination and Autoimmunity - 'vaccinosis': A Dangerous Liaison? ***Journal of Autoimmunity*** 2000;14(1):1-10.
(196) Kerrison J. Optic neuritis after anthrax vaccination. ***Ophthalmology*** 2002;109(1):99-104.
(197) Asatryan A, Pool V, Chen RT, Kohl KS, Davis RL, Iskander JK. Live attenuated measles and mumps viral strain-containing vaccines and hearing loss: Vaccine Adverse Reporting System (VAERS), United States, 1990-2003. ***Vaccine*** 2008;26(8):1166-72.
(186) Roizen NJ. Nongenetic causes of hearing loss. ***Mental Retardation and Developmental Disabilities Research Reviews*** 2003;9(2):120-127
(199) Pickering LK. ***Pediatric News*** November 28, 1998.
(200) Marks AR. Physiological systems under pressure. ***J. Clin. Invest.*** 2008;118(2):411–412.
(201) Sicot C. Medico-Surgical Consultations: ***Le Concours Médical*** 1993;(8)115:
(202) Atkinson W, Hamborsky J, McIntyre L, Wolfe S, eds. (2007). Diphtheria. in: Epidemiology and Prevention of Vaccine-Preventable Diseases (The Pink Book) *(10 ed.). Washington DC: Public Health Foundation. pp. 59–70.*
(203) Biellik RJ, Lobanov A, Heath K, Reichler M, Tjapepua V, Allies T, van Niekerk ABW, Schoub BD. Poliomyelitis in Namibia. ***The Lancet*** 1994;344: 1776.
(204) Gupta N, Puliyel J. WHO study suggests low incidence of Hib in India is due to natural immunity. ***Indian J. Med. Res.*** 2009;129:205-207.
(205) Perry RT, Halsey NA. The Clinical Significance of Measles: A Review. ***The Journal of Infectious Diseases*** 2004;189 (S1):1547-1783.
(206) Manson AL. Mumps orchitis. ***Urology*** *1*990;36 (4):355–8.

(207) Siegel M, Fuerst HT, Guinee VF. Rubella epidemicity and embryopathy. Results of a long-term prospective study. ***Am. J. Dis. Child*** 1971;121(6):469–73.
(208) West R. Epidemiologic study of malignancies of the ovaries. ***Cancer*** 1966;19:1001-1007.
(209) Wynder E, Dodo H, Barber HR. Epidemiology of cancer of the ovary. ***Cancer*** 1969;23:352.
(210) Newhouse M, Pearson RM, Fullerton JM, Boesen EA, Shannon HS. A case control study of carcinoma of the ovary. ***Brit. J. Prev. Soc. Med.*** 1977;31:148-53.
(211) McGowan L, Parent L, Lednar W, Norris HJ. The woman at risk from developing ovarian cancer. ***Gynecol. Oncol.*** 1979;7:325-344.
(212) Kristensen I, Aaby P, Jensen H. Routine vaccinations and child survival: follow-up study in Guinea-Bissau, West Africa. ***British Medical Journal*** 2000;321;1435-9.
(213) Aaby P, Samb B, Simondon F, Coll Seck AM, Knudsen K, Whittle H. Non-specific beneficial effect of measles immunization: analysis of mortality studies from developing countries. ***British Medical Journal*** 1995;311;481-5.
(214) Dalton C, Emerton D, Buckoke C, Finlay R, Engler T, Shann F, Aaby P. Unexpected beneficial effects of measles immunisation. ***British Medical Journal*** 2000;320: 938-938.
(215) Odent MR. Long term effects of early vaccinations. ***Primal Health Research*** 1994;2(1):6.
(216) Polack FP. Why did RSV vaccine make kids sick? ***Nature Medicine*** December 14, 2008.
(217) Quast U, et al. Vaccine-induced mumps-like diseases. ***Developments in Biological Standardization*** 1979;43:269-272.
(218) Ronchi F, Cecchi P, Falcioni F, Marsciani A, Minak G, Muratori G, Tazzari PL, Beverini S. Thrombocytopenic purpura as adverse reaction to recombinant hepatitis B vaccine. ***Archives of Disease in Childhood*** 1998;78(3):273-4.
(219) Tonz O, Bajc S. Convulsions or status epilepticus in 11 infants after pertussis vaccination. ***Schweiz. Med. Wochenschr*** 1980;51:1965-71.
(220) Miller E et al. British Medical Journal 2013. http://www.reuters.com/article/2013/01/31/us-flu-gsk-narcolepsy-britain-idUSBRE90U0JW20130131
(221) Kihei Terada et al. Alterations in Epidemics and vaccination for Measles during a 20 year period and Strategy for Elimination in Kurashiki City, Japan. Kawasaki Medical School 2002;76(3):180-184.
(222) Thompson NP, Montgomery SM, Pounder RE, Wakefield AJ. Is measles vaccination a risk factor for inflammatory bowel disease? ***The Lancet*** 1995;345:1062-3.
(223) Wakefield AJ, Murch SH, Anthony A, Linnell J, Casson DM, Malik M, Berelowitz M, Chillon AP, Thomson MA, Harvey P, Valentine A, Davies SE, Walker-Smith JA. Ileal-lymphoid-nodular hyperplasia, non-specific colitis, and pervasive developmental disorder in children. ***The Lancet*** 1998;351:637-641.
(224) Erickson CA, Stigler KA, Corkins MR, Posey DJ, Fitzgerald JF, McDougle CJ. Gastrointestinal factors in autistic disorder: a critical review. ***J. Autism Dev. Disord.*** 2005; 35(6):713-27.
(225) Fujinaga T, Motegi Y, Tamura H, Kuroume T. A prefecture-wide survey of mumps meningitis associated with MMR vaccine. ***Paediatric Infectious Disease Journal*** (R), March 1991.
(226) Sawada H, Yano S, Oh Y, Togashi T. Transmission of Urabe mumps vaccine between siblings. ***The Lancet*** 1993;342:371.
(227) Adler JB, Mazzotta SA, Barkin JS. Pancreatitis caused by measles, mumps, and rubella vaccine. ***Pancreas*** 1991;6:489-490.
(228) Pawlowski B, Gries FA. Mumps vaccination and type-1 diabetes. ***Deutsche Medizinische Wochenschrift*** 1991;116:635.
(229) Tuomilehto J, Karvonen M, Pitkaniemi J, Virtala E, Kohtamaki K, Toivanen L, Tuomilehto-Wolf E. Record-high incidence of Type I (insulin-dependent) diabetes mellitus in Finnish children. The Finnish Childhood Type I Diabetes Registry Group. ***Diabetologia*** 1999;42(6):655-60.
(230) Weibel RE, Caserta V, Benor DE, Evans G. Acute encephalopathy followed by permanent brain injury or death associated with further attenuated measles vaccines: a review of claims submitted to the National Vaccine Injury Compensation Program. ***Pediatrics*** 1998;101(3), Part 1.
(231) Buttram HE. Measles-Mumps-Rubella (MMR) Vaccine as a Potential Cause of Encephalitis (Brain Inflammation) in Children. ***Townsend Letters***, December 1997.
(232) Laitinen O, Vaheri A. Very high measles and rubella virus antibody titers associated with hepatitis, systemic lupus erythematosus and infectious mononucleosis. ***The Lancet*** 1974;(1):194-7.
(233) Zecca T, Grafino D. Elevated rubeola titers in autistic children linked to MMR vaccine, abstract submitted to the National Institutes of Health, 1997-8.
(234) Halsey NA. Increased mortality after high titer measles vaccine. ***Paediatric Infectious Disease Journal*** (R), June 1993.
(235) Bonthius D, Stanek N, Grose C. Subacute sclerosing panencephalitis, a measles complication, in an internationally adopted child. ***Emerg. Infect. Dis.*** 2000; 6 (4):377–81.
(236) Salmi AA, Norrby E, Panelius M. Identification of different measles virus-specific antibodies in the serum and cerebrospinal fluid from patients with subacute sclerosing pancencephalitis and multiple sclerosis. ***Infect. Immun.*** 1972;6(3):248–254.

(237) Chantler JK, Tingle AJ, Petty RE. Persistent Rubella Virus Associated with Chronic Arthritis in Children. ***N. Engl. J. Med.*** 1985;313(18):117-1123.
(238) Geier MR, Geier DA. A one year followup of chronic arthritis following rubella and hepatitis B vaccination based upon analysis of the Vaccine Adverse Events Reporting System (VAERS) database. ***Clin. Exp. Rheumatol.*** 2002;20(6):767-71.
(239) Bosma TJ, Etherington J, O'Shea S, Corbett K, Cottam F, Holt L, Banatvala JE, Best JM. Rubella Virus and Chronic Joint Disease: Is There an Association? ***J. Clin. Microbiol.*** 1998;36:3524-3526.
(240) Geier MR, Geier DA. Anthrax vaccination and joint related adverse reactions in light of biological warfare scenarios. ***Clin. Exp. Rheumatol.*** 2002;20(1):119.
(241) Geier MR, Geier DA. Arthritic reactions following hepatitis B vaccination: an analysis of the vaccine adverse events reporting system (VAERS) data from 1990 through 1997. ***Clin. Exp. Rheumatol.*** 2000;18(6):789-90.
(242) Ekanem E. A 10 year Review of Morbidity from Childhood Preventable Diseases in Nigeria: How Successful is the Expanded Programe of Immunisation (EPI)? ***J. Tropical Pediatrics*** 1988;34(6):323-8.
(243) McDonald KL, Huq SI, Lix LM, Becker AB, Kozyrskyj AL. Delay in diphtheria, pertussis, tetanus vaccination is associated with a reduced risk of childhood asthma. ***J Allergy Clin. Immunol.*** 2008;121(3):626-31.
(244) Ronne T. Measles virus infection without rash in childhood is related to disease in adult life. ***The Lancet*** 1985; 1(8419):1-5.
(245) Albonico H, Klein P, Grob C, en Pewsner D. The immunization campaign against measles, mumps and rubella -- coercion leading to a realm of uncertainty: medical objections to a continued MMR immunization campaign in Switzerland. *JAMA* 1992; 9(1).
(246) Strebel PM, Aubert-Combiescu A, Ion-Nedelcu N, Biberi-Moroeanu S, Combiescu M, Sutter RW, Kew OM, Pallansch MA, Patriarca PA, Cochi SL. Paralytic poliomyelitis in Romania, 1984-1992. Evidence for a high risk of vaccine-associated disease and reintroduction of wild-virus infection. ***Am. J. Epidemiol.*** 1994;140(12):1111-24.
(247) D'Arcy PF. Vaccine-drug interactions. ***Drug Intelligence & Clinical Pharmacy*** 1984;18(9): 697-700.
(248) Wright SW, Decker MD, Edwards KM. Incidence of pertussis infection in healthcare workers. ***Infect. Control Hosp. Epidemiol.*** 1999;20:120-3.
(249) De Serres G, Bouliane N, Douville Fradet M, Duval B. Pertussis in Quebec: ongoing epidemic since the late 1980s. ***Can. Commun. Dis. Rep.*** 1995;21:45-8.
(250) Andrews R, Herceq A, Roberts C. Pertussis notifications in Australia. ***Commun. Dis. Intell.*** 1997;21:145-8.
(251) Simon MW. Resurgence of Disease in a Highly Immunized Population of Children. ***N. Engl. J. Med.*** 1994;331:16-21.
(252) Markowitz LE, Preblud SR, Orenstein WA, Rovira EZ, Adams NC, Hawkins CE & Hinman AR. Patterns of transmission in measles outbreaks in the United States, 1985-1986. ***N. Engl. J. Med.*** 1989;320:75-81.
(253) Yeung LF, Lurie P, Dayan G, Eduardo E, Britz PH, Redd S.B, Papania MJ, Seward JF. A Limited Measles Outbreak in a Highly Vaccinated US Boarding School. ***Pediatrics*** 2005;116:1287-1291.
(254) Egemen A, Tasdemir I, Eker L, Arcasoy M. Changing Epidemiology of Measles in Turkey: Need for Reassessment of Measles Vaccination Policy? ***J. Trop. Pediatr.*** 1996;42(5):299-301.
(255) Coetzee N, Hussey GD, Visser G, Barron P, Keen A. The 1992 measles epidemic in Cape Town – a changing epidemiological pattern. ***S. Afr. Med. J.***.1994;84(3):145-9.
(256) Gustafson TL, Lievens AW. Brunell PA, Moellenberg,RG. Buttery CMG, Sehulster LM. Measles Outbreak in a Fully Immunised Secondary School Population. New England Journal of Medicine 1987;316(13):771-4.
(257) Miller NZ. Vaccine safety Manual 2008, pp140. Pub. NA Press, Santa Fe.
(258) Cieslak PR. Chickenpox Outbreak in a Highly Vaccinated School Population. Pediatrics 2004;3:455-459
(259) MMWR May 26, 2006 pp559-563.
(260) Schmitt HJ, Wirsing von Konig CH, Neiss A. Efficacy of acellular pertussis vaccine in early childhood after household exposure. *JAMA* 1996; 275:37-41.
(261) Gustafsson L, Hallander HO, Olin P, Reizenstein E, Storsaeter J. A controlled trial of a two-component acellular, a five-component acellular, and a whole-cell pertussis vaccine. ***N. Engl. J. Med.*** 1996;334:349-55.
(262) Briss PA, Fehrs LJ, Parker LA, Wright PF, Sannella EC, Hutcheson RH, Schaffner W. Sustained transmission of mumps in a highly vaccinated population: assessment of vaccine failure and waning vaccine-induced immunity. ***Journal of Infectious Diseases*** 1994; 169:77-82.
(263) Ströhle A, Eggenberger K, Steiner CA, Matter L, Germann D. Mumps epidemic in vaccinated children in West Switzerland. ***Schweiz Med. Wochenschr.*** 1997;127(26):1124-33.
(264) Tayil SE, El-Shazly MK, El-Amrawy SM, Ghouneim FM, Abou Khatwa SA & Masoud GM. Sero-epidemiological study of measles after 15 years of compulsory vaccination in Alexandria, Egypt. ***East Mediterr. Health J.*** 1998;4(3):437-47.
(265) Krause PJ, Cherry JD, Deseda-Tous J, Champion JG, Strassburg M, Sullivan C, Spencer MJ, Byson YJ, Welliver RC, Boyer KM. Epidemic measles in young adults. Clinical, epidemiologic, and serologic studies. ***Ann. Intern. Med.*** 1979;90(6):873-6.

(266) Matter L, Bally F, Germann D, Schopfer K. The incidence of rubella virus infections in Switzerland after the introduction of the MMR Mass vaccination programme. ***European Journal of Epidemiology*** 1995;11(3):305-10.
(267) Alexander LN, Seward JF, Santibanez TA, Pallansch MA Kew OM, Prevots DR, Strebel PM, Cono J, Wharton M, Orenstein WA, Sutter RW. Vaccine Policy Changes and Epidemiology of Poliomyelitis in the United States. ***JAMA*** 2004;292:1696-1701.
(268) Ramsay ME, McVernon J, Andrews NJ, Heath PT, Slack MP. Estimating Haemophilus influenzae type b vaccine effectiveness in England and Wales by use of the screening method. ***J. Infect. Dis.*** 2003;188(4):481-5.
(269) Sarangi J, Cartwright K, Stuart J, Brookes S, Morris R, Slack M. Invasive Haemophilus influenzae disease in adults. ***Epidemiol. Infect.*** 2000;124(3):441-7.
(270) McQuillan GM, Coleman PJ, Kruszon-Moran D, Moyer LA, Lambert SB, Margolis HS. Prevalence of hepatitis B virus infection in the United States: the National Health and Nutrition Examination Surveys, 1976 through 1994. ***Am. J. Public Health*** 1999; 89: 14-18.
(271) Galil K, Fair E, Mountcastle N, Britz P, Seward J. Younger age at vaccination may increase risk of varicella vaccine failure. ***J. Infect. Dis.*** 2002;186(1):102-5.
(272) Tanaka M, Vitek CR, Pascual B, Bisgard KM, Tate JE, Murphy TV. Trends in Pertussis Among Infants in the United States, 1980-1999. ***JAMA*** 2003;290:2968-2975.
(273) Pebody RG, Andrews N, McMenamin J, Durnall H, Ellis J, Thompson CI, Robertson C, Cottrell S, Smyth B, Zambon M, Moore C, Fleming DM, Watson JM. Vaccine effectiveness of 2011/12 trivalent seasonal influenza vaccine in preventing laboratory-confirmed influenza in primary care in the United Kingdom: evidence of waning intra-seasonal protection. ***Eurosurveillance*** 2013 Jan 31:18(5)
(274) The Bercow Report - A Review of Services for Children and Young People (0-19) with Speech, Language and Communication Needs, pub 17-12-2008. Department for Education and Skills (DfES). ISBN 978-1-84775-211-6.
(275) Kootz JP, Marinelli B, Cohen DJ. Sensory receptor sensitivity in autistic children. ***J. Autism and Dev. Disord.*** 1982;12(2):185-193.
(276) Bell JG, MacKinlay EE, Dick JR, MacDonald DJ, Boyle RM, Glen AC. Essential fatty acids and phospholipase A_2 in autistic spectrum disorders. ***Prostaglandins, Leukotrienes and Essential Fatty Acids*** 2004;71(4):201-204.
(277) Warren RP, Margaretten NC, Foster A. Reduced Natural Killer Cell Activity in Autism. ***Journal of the American Academy of Child and Adolescent Psychiatry*** 1987;26(3): 333-335.
(278) Warren RP, Margaretten NC, Pace NC, Foster A. Immune Abnormalities in Patients with Autism. ***J. Autism and Dev. Disord.*** 1986;16(2):189-197.
(279) Warren RP, Yonk LJ, Burger RA, Cole P, Odell JD, Warren WL, White E, Singh V.K. Deficiency of Suppressor-inducer (CD4+CD45RA+) T Cells in Autism. ***Immunological Investigations*** 1990;19(3):245-251.
(280) Del Giuidce-Asch G, Hollander E. Altered immune function in autism. ***International Journal of Neuropsychiatric Medicine*** 1997;2:61-68.
(281) DeLong GR. Autism: new data suggest a new hypothesis. ***Neurology*** 1999;52(5):911-916.
(282) Cannell JJ. Autism and Vitamin D. ***Medical Hypotheses*** 2008;70(4):750-9.
(283) Coyle P, Philcox JC, Carey LC, Rofe AM. Metallothionine: the multipurpose protein. ***Cellular and Molecular Life Sciences*** 2002;59(4) 627-647.
(284) Maret W. Metallothionein redox biology in the cytoprotective and cytotoxic functions of zinc. ***Experimental Gerontology*** 2008;43(5):363-369.
(285) West CE. Vitamin A and measles. ***Nutr. Rev.*** 2000;58(2 Pt 2):S46-54.
(286) Barclay AJ, Foster A, Sommer A. Vitamin A supplements and mortality related to measles: a randomised clinical trial. ***Br. Med. J. (Clin Res Ed)***1987; 294(6567):294-6.
(287) Filipek PA, Juranek J, Nguyen MT, Cummings C, Gargus JJ. Relative carnitine deficiency in autism. ***J. Autism Dev. Disord.*** 2004;34(6):615-23.
(288) Lake CR, Ziegler MG, Murphy DL. Increased norepinephrine levels and decreased dopamine-hydroxylase activity in primary autism. ***Arch. Gen. Psychiatry*** 1977;34:553-6.
(289) Todd R, Ciaranello R. Demonstration of inter-and intraspecies differences in serotonin binding sites by antibodies from an autistic child. ***Proc. Nat. Acad. Sci.*** 1985;82:612-616.
(290) Bingham M. Autism and the Human Gut Microflora. May 2002
(291) Wakefield AJ, Anthony A, Murch SH, Thomson M, Montgomery SM, Davies S, O'Leary JJ, Berelowitz M, Walker-Smith JA. Enterocolitis in Children with Developmental Disorders. ***Am. J. Gastroenterology*** 2000;95(9):2285-2295.
(292) Stubbs G, Litt M, Lis E, Jackson R, Voth W, Lindberg A, Litt R. Adenosine Deaminase Activity Decreased in Autism. ***J. Am. Acad. Child Psych.*** 1982;21:71-74.
(293) Persico AM, Militerni R, Bravaccio C, Schneider C, Melmed R, Trillo S, Montecchi F, Palermo MT, Pascucci T, Puglisi-Allegra S, Reichelt KL, Conciatori M, Baldi A, Keller F. Adenosine Deaminase Alleles and Autistic Disorder. ***Am. J. Med. Genetics*** 2000;96:784-790.

(294) Torrente FP Ashwood P, Day R, Machado N, Furlano RA, Anthony A, Davies S E, Wakefield AJ, Thomson MA, Walker-Smith JA & Murch SH. Small intestinal enteropathy with epithelial, IgG and complement deposition in children with regressive autism. ***Molec. Psych*** 2002;7:375-382.
(295) Fillano JJ, Goldenthal MJ, Harker Rhodes C, Marin-Garcia J. Mitochondrial dysfunction in patients with hypotonia, epilepsy, autism, and developmental delay: HEADD syndrome. ***J. Child Neurol.*** *2002;*17(6): 435-9.
(296) Oliveira G, Diogo L, Grazina M, Garcia P, Ataide A, Marques C, Miguel T, Borges L, Vicente AM, Oliveira CR. Mitochondrial dysfunction in autism spectrum disorders: a population-based study. ***Dev. Med. Child Neurol.*** 2005;47:185-9.
(297) Niederhofer H, Staffen W, Mair A. Lofexidine In Hyperactive And Impulsive Children With Autistic Disorder. ***Journal of the American Academy of Child & Adolescent Psychiatry*** 2002; 41(12):1396-1397.
(298) Birmaher B, Quintana H, Greenhill LL. Methylphenidate treatment of hyperactive autistic children. ***J. Am. Acad. Child Adol. Psychiatry*** 1988;27:248–251.
(299) Perry R, Campbell M, Adams P, Lyneh N, Speneer EK. Long-term efficacy of haloperidol in autistic children: Continuous versus discontinuous drug administration. ***J. Am. Acad. Child Adolesc. Psychiatry*** 1959;25:57-92.
(300) Cohen DJ, Young JG, Nathanson JA, Shaywitz BA. Clonidine in Tourette's syndrome. ***The Lancet*** 1979;2:551-553.
(301) Niederhofer H, Staffen W, Mair A. Tianeptine: a novel strategy of psychopharmacological treatment of children with autistic disorder. ***Human Psychopharmacology*** 2003;18(5):389-393.
(302) Niederhofer H, Staffen W, Mair A. Galantamine may be effective in treating autistic disorder. ***British Medical Journal*** 2002;325:1422.
(303) Niederhofer H, Staffen W, Mair A. Immunoglobulins as an Alternative Strategy of Psychopharmacological Treatment of Children with Autistic Disorder. ***Neuropsychopharmacology*** 2003;28:1014-1015.
(304) Niederhofer H, Staffen W, Mair A, Pittschieler K. Melatonin facilitates sleep in individuals with mental retardation and insomnia. ***J. Autism Dev. Disord.*** 2003;33(4):469-72.
(305) Ratey JJ, Bemporad J, Sorgi P, Bick P, Polakoff S, O'Driscoll G, Mikkelsen E. Brief report: Open trial effects of beta-blockers on speech and social behaviors in 8 autistic adults. ***Journal of Autism and Dev. Disord.*** 1987;17(3): 439-446.
(306) Beaudet AL. Autism: highly heritable but not inherited. ***Nature Medicine*** 2007;13:534-536.
(307) Jiang YH, Yuen RK, Jin X, Wang M, Chen N, Wu X, Ju J, Mei J, Shi Y, He M, Wang G, Liang J, Wang Z, Cao D, Carter MT, Chrysler C, Drmic IE, Howe JL, Lau L, Marshall CR, Merico D, Nalpathamkalam T, Thiruvahindrapuram B, Thompson A, Uddin M, Walker S, Luo J, Anagnostou E, Zwaigenbaum L, Ring RH, Wang J, Lajonchere C, Wang J, Shih A, Szatmari P, Yang H, Dawson G, Li Y, Scherer SW. 2013. Detection of clinically relevant genetic variants in autism spectrum disorder by whole-genome sequencing. ***Am J Hum Genet***. doi: 10.1016/j.ajhg.2013.06.012.
(308) Dennis EL, Jahanshad N, Rudie JD, Brown JA, Johnson K, McMahon KL, de Zubicaray GI, Montgomery G, Martin NG, Wright MJ, Bookheimer SY, Dapretto M, Toga AW, Thompson PM. Altered structural brain connectivity in healthy carriers of the autism risk gene, CNTNAP2. ***Brain Connect.*** 2012;2(6):356.
(309) Christine Wu Nordahl, Amaral DG, et al. Boys with regressive autism have larger brains than counterparts. ***Proceedings of the National Academy of Sciences*** issue of November 29, 2011.
(310) Richler J, Luyster R, Risi S, Hsu WL, Dawson G, Bernier R, Dunn M, Hepburn S, Hyman SL, McMahon WM, Goudie-Nice J, Minshew N, Rogers S, Sigman M, Spence MA, Goldberg WA, Tager-Flusberg H, Volkmar FR, Lord C. Is there a 'regressive phenotype' of Autism Spectrum Disorder associated with the measles-mumps-rubella vaccine? a CPEA study". ***J. Autism Dev. Disord.*** 2006;36 (3): 299–316.
(311) Matsunami N, Hadley D, Hensel CH, Christensen GB, Kim C, Frackelton E, Thomas K, Pellegrino da Silva R, Stevens J, Baird L, Otterud B, Ho K, Varvil T, Leppert T, Lambert CG, Leppert M, Hakonarson H. Identification of Rare Recurrent Copy Number Variants in High-Risk Autism Families and Their Prevalence in a Large ASD Population. ***PLoS One*** 2013;8(1):e52239. doi: 10.1371/journal.pone.0052239. Epub 2013 Jan 14.
(312) Minshew NJ. 'Brief Report: Brain Mechanisms in Autism: Functional and Structural Abnormalities', ***J. Autism and Dev. Disord.*** 1996;26(2):205-209.
(313) Busto R, Dietrich WD, Globus MY, Valdes I, Scheinberg P, Ginsberg MD. Small differences in intraischemic brain temperature critically determine the extent of ischemic neuronal injury. ***J. Cereb. Blood Flow Metab.*** 1987;7:729–738.
(314) Torres AR. Is fever suppression involved in the etiology of autism and neurodevelopmental disorders? ***BMC Pediatr.*** 2003;3:9.
(315) Urnovitz HB, Tuite JJ, Higashida JM, Murphy WH. RNAs in the Sera of Persian Gulf War Veterans Have Segments Homologous to Chromosome 22q11.2.***Clinical and Diagnostic Laboratory Immunology*** 1999;6(3):330-335.
(316) Rook GAW, Zumla A. Gulf War Syndrome: is it due to a systemic shift in cytokine balance towards Th2 profile? ***The Lancet*** 1997;349;1831-3.
(317) Meggs WJ. Multiple Chemical Sensitivities and the Immune System. ***Tox. Indust. Health*** 1994;8:203-214.

(318) Hotopf M, David A, Hull L, Ismail K, Unwin C, Wessely S. Role of Vaccinations as risk factors for ill health in veterans of the Gulf War: cross sectional study. ***British Medical Journal*** 2000;320;1363-7.

(319) Hou L, Zhang X, Wang D, Baccarelli A. Environmental chemical exposures and human epigenetics. ***Int. J. Epidemiol.*** (2012) 41 (1): 79-105. doi: 10.1093/ije/dyr154

(320) Monks TJ, Xie R, Tikoo K, Lau SS. Ros-induced histone modifications and their role in cell survival and cell death. ***Drug Metab. Rev.*** 2006;38(4):755-67.

(321) Hemdan NY, Emmrich F, Faber S, Lehmann J, Sack U. Alterations of TH1/TH2 reactivity by heavy metals: possible consequences include induction of autoimmune diseases. ***Ann. NY Acad. Sci.*** 2007 Aug;1109:129-37.

(322) Pilsner JR, Lazarus AL, Nam DH, et al. Mercury-associated DNA hypomethylation in polar bear brains via the LUminometric Methylation Assay: a sensitive method to study epigenetics in wildlife. ***Mol. Ecol.*** *2010;19:307-14.*

(323) Arai Y, Ohgane J, Yagi S, et al. Epigenetic Assessment of environmental chemicals detected in maternal peripheral and cord blood samples. ***J. Reprod. Dev.*** 2011;57:507-17.

(324) Pogue AI, Li YY, Cui JG, et al. Characterization of an NF-kappaB-regulated, miRNA-146a-mediated down-regulation of complement factor H (CFH) in metal-sulfate-stressed human brain cells. ***J. Inorg. Biochem.*** 2009;103:1591-95.

(325) Lukiw WJ, Pogue AI. Induction of specific micro RNA (miRNA) species by ROS-generating metal sulfates in primary human brain cells. ***J. Inorg. Biochem.*** 2007;101:1265-69.

(326) DeSoto MC. Blood Levels of Mercury Are Related to Diagnosis of Autism: A Reanalysis of an Important Data Set. ***Journal of Child Neurology*** 2007;22(11):1308-1311.

(327) Tokuomi H. Uchino M. Imamura S. Yamanaga H. Nakanishi R. Ideta T. Minamata disease (organic mercury poisoning): Neuroradiologic and electrophysiologic studies. ***Neurology*** 1982;32:1369-1375.

(328) Palmer RF, Blanchard S, Stein Z, Mandell D, Miller C. Environmental mercury release, special education rates, and autism disorder: an ecological study of Texas. ***Health & Place*** 2006;12(2): 203-209.

(329) Amin-Zaki L, Majeed MA, Clarkson TW, Greenwood MR. Methylmercury poisoning in Iraqi children: clinical observations over two years. ***British Medical Journal*** 1978 March 1, 613-616.

(330) Joselow MW, Louria DB, Browder AA. Mercurialism: Environmental and occupational aspects. ***Annals of Internal Medicine*** 1972;76:119-30.

(331) Wecker L, Miller S.B, Cochran SR, Dugger DL, Johnson WD. Trace Element Concentrations in Hair From Autistic Children. ***J. Ment. Defic. Res.*** 1985;29:15-22.

(332) Adams CR, Ziegler DK, Lin JT. Mercury intoxication simulating amyotrophic lateral sclerosis. ***JAMA*** 1983; 250:642-643.

(333) Fagala GE, Wigg CL. Psychiatric manifestations of mercury poisoning. ***J. Am. Acad. Child Adolesc. Psychiatry*** 1992;31(2):306-311.

(334) Kark RAP, Poskanzer DC, Bullock JD, Boylen G. Mercury poisoning and its treatment with n-acetyl-d, l-penicillamine. ***N. Engl. J. Med.***1971;285:10-16.

(335) Teitelbaum P, Teitelbaum O, Nye J, Fryman J, Maurer RG. Movement Analysis in infancy may be useful for early diagnosis of autism. ***PNAS*** 1998;95(23):13982-13987.

(336) Church C, Coplan J. The high functioning autistic experience: Birth to pre-teen years. ***J. Pediatric Health Care*** 1995;9(22):29.

(337) Makani S, Gollapudi S, Yel L, Chiplunkar S, Gupta S. Biochemical and molecular basis of thimerosal-induced apoptosis in T-cells: a major role of mitochondrial pathway. **Genes and Immunity** 2002;3:270-278.

(338) Shenker BJ, Datar S, Mansfield K, Shapiro IM. Induction of apoptosis in human T-cells by organomercuric compounds: a flow dytometric analysis. ***Toxicol. Appl. Pharmacol.*** 1997;143(2):397-406.

(339) Yonk LJ, Warren KP, Burger RA, Cote P, Odell JD, Warren WL, White E, Singh VK. CD4 helper –T cell depletion in autism. ***Immunology Letters*** 1990;25:344-346.

(340) Parker SK, Schwartz B, Todd J, Pickering LK. Thimerosal-Containing Vaccines and Autistic Spectrum Disorder: A Critical Review of Published Original Data. ***Pediatrics*** 2004;114(3):793-804.

(341) Madsen KM, Lauritsen MB, Pedersen CB, Thorsen P, Plesner A-M, Andersen PH, Mortensen PB. Thimerosal and the Occurrence of Autism: Negative Ecological Evidence From Danish Population-Based Data. ***Pediatrics*** 2003;112(3):604-606.

(342) DeSoto MC, Hitlan RT. Relationship between mercury and autism - autistic children may be less efficient at eliminating mercury from the blood. ***J. Child Neurol.***.2007;22: 1308-11.

(343) Kabuto M. Chronic effects of methylmercury on the urinary excretion of catecholamines and their responses to hypoglycemic stress. ***Arch. Toxical.*** 1991; 65(2):164-167.

(344) http://www.merck.com/mmpe/sec13/ch164/ch164a.html

(345) Clarkson TW. Mercury: major issues in environmental health. ***Environ. Health Perspect.*** 1992; 100: 31-38.

(346) Brenner RP, Snyder RD. Late EEG finding and clinical status after organic mercury poisoning. ***Arch. Neurol.*** 1980; 37(5): 282-284.

(347) Grandjean P, Weihe P, White RF, Debes F. Cognitive performance of children prenatally exposed to 'safe' levels of methylmercury. ***Environmental Research*** 1998;77(2):165-172.

(348) Rice DC, Gilbert SG. Early chronic low-level methylmercury poisoning in monkeys impairs spatial vision. ***Science*** 1982;216(4547):759-761.
(349) Counter SA, Buchanan LH. Mercury exposure in children: a review. ***Toxicology and Applied Pharmacology*** 2004;198(2):209-230.
(350) Hrdina PD, Peters DA, Singhal RL. Effects of chronic exposure to cadmium, lead and mercury of brain biogenic amines in the rat. ***Research Communications in Chemistry, Pathology and Pharmacology*** 1976;15(3):483-493.
(351) Flarend RE, Hem SL. In vivo absorption of aluminum-containing vaccine adjuvants using 26Al. ***Vaccine*** 1997;15:1314-1318.
(352) Sharpe MA, Gist TL, Baskin DS. B-Lymphocytes from a population of Children with Autistic Spectrum Disorder and their Unaffected Siblings exhibit Hypersensitivity to Thimerosal. Journal of Toxicology submitted 2013.
(353) Rimland B. Recovery from autism is possible. ***Autism Research Review International*** 1994;8(2):3.
(354) Rimland B, Baker S.M. Brief Report: Alternative Approaches to the Development of Effective Treatments for Autism. ***J. Autism and Dev. Disord.*** 1996;26(2):237-241.
(355) Rossignol D, Rossignol L. Hyperbaric oxygen therapy may improve symptoms in autistic children. ***Medical Hypotheses*** 2006;67(2):216-228.
(356) Lavine L. Osteopathic and Alternative Medicine Aspects of Autistic Spectrum Disorders. ***First International Autism Internet Conference, British Autism Society***, London, England (1999).
(357) Jarusiewicz B. Efficacy of neurofeedback for children in the autistic spectrum: A pilot study. ***Journal of Neurotherapy*** 2002;6(4):39-49.
(358) Kouijzer MEUJ, de Moor JMH, Gerrits BJL, Buitelaar JK, van Schie HT. Long-term effects of neurofeedback treatment in autism. ***Research in Autism Spectrum Disorders*** 2009;3:496-501.
(359) Sichel AG, Fehmi LG, Goldstein DM. Positive outcome with neurofeedback treatment of a case of mild autism. ***Journal of Neurotherapy*** 1995;1(1):60-64.
(360) Levy SE, Hyman SL. Novel Treatments for Autistic Spectrum Disorders ***Mental Retardation and Developmental Disabilities Research Reviews*** 2005;11:131-142.
(361) Sommer A, Katz J, Tarwotjo I. Increased risk of respiratory disease and diarrhea in children with pre-existing vitamin A deficiency. ***Am. J. Clin. Nutr.*** 1984;40:1090-5.
(362) Kang D-W, Park JG, Ilhan ZE, Wallstrom G, LaBaer J, et al. Reduced Incidence of *Prevotella* and Other Fermenters in Intestinal Microflora of Autistic Children. ***PLoS ONE*** 2013;8(7):e68322. doi:10.1371/journal.pone.0068322
(363) Campbell-McBride N. http://www.gaps.me/?page_id=20
(364) Weber W, Newmark S . Complementary and alternative medical therapies for attention-deficit/hyperactivity disorder and autism. ***Pediatr. Clin. North Am.*** 2007;54 (6): 983–1006.
(365) Gustafson TL, Lievens AW, et al. Measles outbreak in a fully immunized secondary-school population. ***N. Engl. J. Med.*** 1987;316(13):771-4.
(366) Thompson J. Vaccine antibodies are lower in very premature babies. ***Community Practitioner*** April 1, 2002.
(367) http://www.dyslexia-international.org/Educational%20Authorities/About%20dyslexia%20ea
(368) http://www.bbc.co.uk/news/uk-scotland-24206322

Over many years of doing in research in autism spectrum disorder, I have had the opportunity to talk with many parents. Most have reported that their child was normal until a vaccine or vaccines. Their voices are brushed aside by the experts and authorities stating that the parents are wrong. The voice that overshadows the voice of the parents, for the most part, is the US Centers for Disease Control and Prevention (CDC). The CDC states publicly that there is no relationship between vaccines and autism, and that Thimerosal, a mercury-based preservative used in vaccines, could not cause the symptoms seen in autism. However, their internal documents tell a completely different story. The internal documents make clear that they will not say in public what they know in private because they are worried about the vaccine program and potential lawsuits. Many scientists and researchers shy away from the topic because it is controversial. Consequently, there are few left to give voice the parents and children. This book, written by Graham Ewing is a voice for the parents and children. He is a scientist who is willing to be true to the science and face an issue that so many steer away from. He has the courage to face the issue and to write publicly about it, and for that, I am very grateful.

Janet Kern, PhD.

www.ingramcontent.com/pod-product-compliance
Ingram Content Group UK Ltd.
Pitfield, Milton Keynes, MK11 3LW, UK
UKHW021332070726
13610UKWH00011B/35